Tasks for Part 3 MRCOG Clinical Assessment

Tasks for Part 3 MRCOG Clinical Assessment

Edited by

Sambit Mukhopadhyay
Consultant
Norfolk and Norwich University Hospital Foundation Trust, Norwich, UK

and

Medha Sule
Consultant
Norfolk and Norwich University Hospital Foundation Trust, Norwich, UK

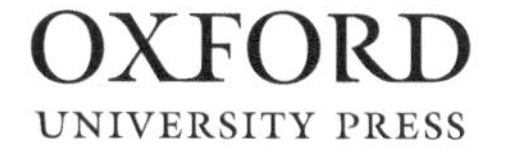
OXFORD
UNIVERSITY PRESS

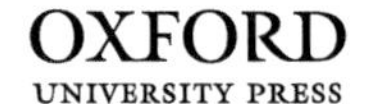

Great Clarendon Street, Oxford, OX2 6DP,
United Kingdom

Oxford University Press is a department of the University of Oxford.
It furthers the University's objective of excellence in research, scholarship,
and education by publishing worldwide. Oxford is a registered trade mark of
Oxford University Press in the UK and in certain other countries

First Edition published in 2018

Published in the United States of America by Oxford University Press
198 Madison Avenue, New York, NY 10016, United States of America

British Library Cataloguing in Publication Data
Data available

Library of Congress Control Number: 2017941747

ISBN 978–0–19–875712–2

Printed and bound by
CPI Group (UK) Ltd, Croydon, CR0 4YY

Foreword

The new MRCOG examination has three parts. Part I examination on basic sciences in early years of training. This is followed by the Part 2 examination after few years of training. Part 2 consists of single best answer (SBAs) questions and extended matching questions (EMQs). Passing the MRCOG Part 3 would determine whether one could proceed to become a specialist. Part 3 assesses the candidate's ability to apply one's core knowledge, skills and attitude to a given clinical situation relevant to daily clinical practise. The candidate should have adequate knowledge in the subject of obstetrics and gynaecology (O&G), good communications skills and attitude that takes into consideration the sociocultural issues of various communities in the UK in addition to organisational issues. The care given should be patient centred, safe, and of the expected quality based on available evidence based guidelines. The book *Tasks for Part 3 MRCOG Clinical Assessment* by Drs Sambit Mukhopadhyay and Medha Sule is one of the best books available for improving your knowledge and practise in these areas to get maximum marks in the Part 3 clinical assessment examination.

This book has 20 chapters consisting of 79 clinical assessment tasks covering the span of O&G ('blue printing') that is needed to pass the examination. The number of questions in each chapter varies based on the breadth and depth of the knowledge needed and the tasks are examples in the different areas. The chapters are written by authors well recognised in their area of special interest and who have number of years of clinical experience and who have participated in training or examining for the MRCOG examination. Each question gives detailed instructions to the candidate, role player and the examiner/assessor. The examination evaluates the patient safety; communication with patients and their relatives; communication with colleagues; information gathering, and applied clinical knowledge. The marking is graded as pass, borderline, or fail. With each task, notes are provided to the candidates to enhance their knowledge on that topic in addition to tips to enhance their performance. By practising these tasks, it will become clear that counselling is not mere communication. Suitable information is provided about additional reading mainly in the form of guidelines from the RCOG and other relevant bodies. This should encourage further learning by the candidate.

I would strongly recommend the *Tasks for Part 3 MRCOG Clinical Assessment* as essential reading for those who appear for the Part 3 MRCOG examination. More importantly, I encourage you practise these tasks with your peers in an examination like environment to maximally benefit from this excellent book.

Best wishes to all candidates for the examination.

S Arulkumaran
Past President of the RCOG ('07-'10), BMA ('13-'14), FIGO ('12-'15)
2017

Preface

In the UK the MRCOG exam is the exit examination from intermediate training. The aim of the examination is to assess core competencies in knowledge, skills, and attitudes as defined in the curriculum. The clinical assessment tasks part of Part 2 is uncoupled and is introduced as a standalone new Part 3 clinical assessment examination. The MRCOG is an UK exam taken globally. In many countries MRCOG exam is considered as a specialist qualification and a licence to independent specialist practice.

In our day-to-day medicine we seldom practise pure science but applied knowledge relevant to a clinical context. Diseases and illnesses have to be viewed in the societal context and therefore methods of assessment for competencies reflect the cultural and organisational nuances of society. The new Part 3 clinical assessment aims to assess candidates' ability to apply core knowledge, skills, and attitudes relevant to the day to day UK clinical practice. This book provides over 75 clinical assessment tasks drawn from day-to-day clinical settings. We have included detailed instructions for role player for each station which we believe will give a greater insight to candidates. This will enable them to be aware of the psychosocial issues related to clinical presentation. For overseas trainees who are not exposed to the UK system this book will help to address some aspects of cultural and organisational nuances.

Information gathering and giving are the fundamental skills required for safe clinical practice. We have included a separate chapter on communication skills focusing on initiation of patient centred consultation based on Cambridge-Calgary model. We believe this will provide a framework for developing good communication skills particularly for overseas candidates who practices medicine in a different socio-cultural environment.

We have endeavoured to cover the curriculum as widely as possible to give a flavour of this examination. We must stress that the candidates should be up-to-date with the most recently published guidelines published by the Royal College of Obstetricians and Gynaecologists.

Self-assessment is an important tool for the preparation of any examinations. Immediate peer feedback to the candidate will help to hone skills required to be successful in clinical tasks. Furthermore, the book also provides reference for further reading to improve the knowledge base. We believe that this practical guide to Part 3 MRCOG will be invaluable to trainees all over the world who are preparing to take the Part 3 Membership Examination of the Royal College of Obstetricians and Gynaecologists.

Finally, it would not have been possible to develop this book without help of the contributors for this book who have worked tirelessly to develop these questions. They have been chosen from senior trainees to specialists who are full time clinicians and actively involved in medical education, training and assessment. We are grateful to all of them and express our sincere thanks for giving up their valuable time to develop this book.

Sambit Mukhopadhyay
Medha Sule
2017

Contents

Contributors

PS Arunakumari, Consultant Gynaecologist, Norfolk and Norwich University Hospital Foundation Trust, Norwich, UK.

Maya Basu, Consultant Obstetrician and Gynaecologist and Subspecialist in Urogynaecology, Rochester, UK.

Miriam Baumgarten, Consultant in Reproductive Medicine and Surgery, Cambridge University Hospitals Foundation Trust, Cambridge, UK.

Eamonn Breslin, Consultant Maternal Fetal Medicine at Leicester, Leicester, Leicestershire, UK.

Charlotte Cassis, Clinical Research Fellow, Norfolk and Norwich University Hospital NHS Trust, Norwich, UK.

Mausumi Das, Consultant Gynaecologist and Obstetrician, Nottingham City Hospital, NHS Trust, UK.

Jo Evans, Consultant in Genito Urinary Medicine, Department/Service: iCaSH Norwich, Norfolk, UK.

Ilias Giarenis, Consultant Gynaecologist, Norfolk and Norwich University Hospital Foundation Trust, Norwich, UK.

Sonal Grover, Speciality Trainee, Norfolk and Norwich University Hospital, Foundation Trust, UK.

Anna Haestier, Consultant Obstetrician, Norfolk and Norwich University Hospital Foundation Trust, Norwich, UK.

Manjiri Khare, Consultant Maternal-Fetal Medicine at Leicester, Leicester, Leicestershire, UK.

Milind Kulkarni, Consultant Paediatric Surgeon, Norfolk and Norwich University Hospital NHS Trust, Norwich, UK.

Bidyut Kumar, Consultant Obstetrician and Gynaecologist, Betsi Cadwalader University Health Board, UK.

Geeta Kumar, Clinical Director, Women's Services (East), BCUHB and Consultant Obstetrician and Gynaecologist, Betsi Cadwala University Health Board, UK.

Neeraja Kuruba, Consultant Gynaecologist, Norfolk and Norwich University Hospital Foundation Trust, Norwich, UK.

Jane MacDougall, Consultant in Reproductive Medicine and Surgery, Cambridge University Hospitals Foundation Trust, Cambridge, UK.

Edward Morris, Consultant Gynaecologist, Norfolk and Norwich University Foundation Trust, Norwich, UK.

Sambit Mukhopadhyay, Consultant Gynaecologist, Norfolk and Norwich University NHS Trust, Norwich, UK.

Saadia Naeem, Locum consultant Obstetrician and Gynaecologist, James Paget Hospital NHS Trust, Great Yarmouth, UK.

Asma Naqi, Clinical Teaching Fellow, Department of Obstetrics and Gynaecology, Norfolk and Norwich University Hospital NHS Trust, Norwich, UK.

Gemma Partridge, Speciality trainee, East of England Deanery, UK.

Alka Prakash, Consultant in Reproductive Medicine and Surgery, Cambridge University Hospitals Foundation Trust, Cambridge, UK.

Sarah Prince, Speciality trainee, East of England Deanery, UK.

Catherine Schunmann, Consultant in Sexual and Reproductive Health, Integrated Contraception and Sexual Health for Cambridgeshire Community Services NHS Trust, Cambridge, UK.

Medha Sule, Consultant Gynaecologist, Norfolk and Cambridge University Hospitals Foundation Trust, UK.

Hilary Turnbull, Consultant Gynaecological Oncologist, Norfolk and Norwich University Hospital Foundation Trust, Norwich, UK.

Rachel Wamboldt, medical student, Norwich Medical School, University of East Anglia, Norwich, UK.

Introduction

How to use this book?

The Part 2 MRCOG Clinical assessment is now uncoupled from the written examination and is introduced as a standalone Part 3 clinical assessment examination or more popularly known as Part 3 MRCOG. The aim of the examination is to assess candidates' ability to apply core clinical skills in the context of skills knowledge, attitudes and competencies as defined in the curriculum. The clinical assessment exam is blueprinted distinctly from the written exam with specific emphasis on oral specific domains. Candidates who pass the Part 2 MRCOG written examination must attempt the Part 3 MRCOG clinical assessment within seven years. All candidates (UK based and overseas) are permitted four attempts at the new Part 3 MRCOG clinical assessment. If they are unsuccessful within four attempts they will be required to retake Part 2 MRCOG. For regulations in examination currency and number of attempts please visit the RCOG website.

Part 3 Clinical Assessment

Part 3 MRCOG comprises a circuit of 14, 12 (including 2 minutes reading time) minute stations, in which each candidate is examined on a one-to-one basis with one examiner and simulated (role players) patients. There is no preparatory station in the current format. Candidates rotate through the stations, completing all the stations on their circuit. In this way, all candidates take the same stations and the total duration of the exam is 168 minutes. Tasks in the stations are aligned to 14 modules of the curriculum, and assessment is designed on the basis of five core skills of good medical practice. These are patient safety, communicating with patient and families, communicating with colleagues, information gathering, and applied clinical knowledge. Each task will assess number of these domains.

Preparation

Preparing for clinical assessment tasks is very different from preparing for an examination on theory. In these tasks, core clinical skills and application of knowledge are tested rather than pure theoretical knowledge. There is a great emphasis on assessment of communication skills in the context of a particular clinical situation. It is not about what you know about a particular task but how you present the information. Therefore, it is essential to practice repeatedly until you have honed the art of information gathering and giving. This book provides a wide curriculum coverage with example of clinical assessment tasks drawn from all the modules of the curriculum. Collaborative learning and practicing these tasks with a friend relieves the stress and boredom. We learn from each other's strengths and weaknesses and more importantly it disciplines you and keeps you on track to achieve your goals. We recommend you to practise in small groups with colleagues, selecting a typical clinical assessment task, and timing it with one person acting as a patient, one person performing the task and if possible, a third person examining and providing feedback using mark sheet provided with each task. By doing this you will be able to get a feel of 'running to time' and working under pressure.

In keeping with the MRCOG 3 clinical assessment, we have included the domains of: patient safety, communication with patients and their relatives, communication with colleagues, information gathering, and applied clinical knowledge in sample mark sheets throughout the book. These are aligned to the GMC's good medical practice. We therefore believe that practising these tasks in the structured format provided will enable you to cover competencies demanded in all domains of good medical practice required by the General Medical Council. We have also included a separate chapter on communication skills.

The ability to pass or fail in a high stake examination depends on an acceptable level of competencies set by the examination board. The ability to communicate and to apply knowledge to solve clinical problems to ensure safety and quality in the UK clinical practice form the core of Part 3 MRCOG. In your day-to-day practice it is useful to covert some clinical encounters (e.g. checking scan and HCG results in the Early Pregnancy Unit) to potential mini clinical assessment tasks and think of possible questions and rehearse. Examination can be stressful and nerve-wracking but the more you practice less the fear and stress on the day. With over 75 tasks and wide curriculum coverage, this book will provide you with ample opportunities to practice and address areas where you may want to improve. Keep practising....

Further reading

https://www.rcog.org.uk/en/careers-training/mrcog-exams/regulations-on-mrcog-exam-currency-and-number-of-attempts/.

Chapter 1 **Communication skills and tips for Part 3 MRCOG examination**

Good communication skills form a fundamental principle of the patient-centred clinical consultation. The new Part 3 of the MRCOG, assesses candidates based on their ability to apply the core clinical skills in the context of real-life scenarios. It assesses five core skills domains, with three relating to communication skills; i) Communicating with patients and their families, ii) Communicating with colleagues and iii) Information gathering.

Communication skills in the Part 3 clinical assessment can be assessed in many forms:

- Exploring patient symptoms or concerns (information gathering)
- Explaining a diagnosis, investigation or treatment (information giving)
- Involving the patient in a decision (shared decision making)
- Health promoting activities
- Obtaining informed consent for a procedure
- Breaking bad news
- Communicating with relatives
- Communicating with other members of the health care team

In order to provide patient-centred care, doctors must treat their patients as partners, involving them in the decision making regarding their care and instilling in them a sense of responsibility for their own health. When the patient feels that they are part of the team it increases their satisfaction with care, increases treatment adherence and improves clinical outcomes. It is these skills that are assessed in clinical assessment tasks involving communication.

Clinical assessment candidates are often assessed in two communication domains; Process and Content. In order to do well in the information gathering stations, you must be aware of the differential diagnoses that may arise with various presentations and how to explore each one independently and as a collection. When it comes to information giving or shared decision marking, candidates need to be familiar with the most recent Royal College of Obstetrics and Gynaecology guidelines and know how to interpret their meaning to the patient and their families.

The Calgary-Cambridge Model is one of the most recognized communication theories in medical education (Kurtz, 1996). This theory can be adapted to fit into most clinical scenarios. Using the Calgary-Cambridge Model, you should be able to obtain the majority of the points related to process. The five communication skills principles of the model that are also assessed in clinical assessment include:

1. Initiating the session
2. Gathering information
3. Building the relationship
4. Explanation and planning
5. Closing the session

Step-by-Step guide for achieving process points

Preparation and composure before entering the clinical assessment task is critical for success. Take time to read the vignette carefully, taking note of what is expected from you in the station—information gathering versus information giving. Clinical information can be checked with the patient if you forget certain details, but misinterpreting the purpose (task) of the station can set you up for a disaster. You are not required to enter the station as soon as you are instructed to. If you need slightly more time to gather your thoughts, do so before entering. Roger Neighbour referred to this as 'housekeeping' (2004).

Initiating the session

- First impressions are crucial. Enter the station slowly and confidently making eye contact with the patient and smiling
- Start with a generic greeting, such as 'Good morning' and then introduce yourself, your role and the purpose of consultation
- Confirm that you have the correct patient by asking for their name and age
- Ask an open question to start the consultation. This is often a matter of personal choice but, 'How can I help you today?' will suffice
- The golden minute is an opportunity for the patient to explain in their own words the reason for the consultation. Do not interrupt the patient until they are finished. Use active listening skills to encourage the patient to tell you more
    - Active listening techniques include nodding, reflective facial expressions and continued eye contact. Neutral verbal cues can also be used such as "uh-huh', 'yes', and 'I see'. This lets the patient know that you are interested and concerned about what they are telling you (Tongue, 2005)
- When the patient has completed their initial narrative. Acknowledge any emotions that they might have expressed by saying, 'I'm sorry that you have been feeling this way' or something similar
- It is useful at this stage to summarize what the patient has said in order to give yourself time to think about how to proceed
- Before moving forward, screen for any hidden agendas with a question like, 'Is there anything else that you were hoping to discuss today?'
- Agenda setting is a very important part of initiating the session. Signpost to the patient that you would like to ask more specific questions about why they have come in today

Gathering information

The purpose of this stage of the consultation is to explore the issue at hand and to determine the patient's perspective (Kurtz, 1996).

- Based on the presenting features in the Golden Minute, begin to ask focused questions. Start with open questions such as 'Can you tell me a bit more about the bleeding?' Then narrow your questioning down to determine specific details (e.g. 'Do you experience bleeding during or after sexual activity?'). Closed questions should only be used to fill in the gaps (Fernando, 2011)
- Each symptom needs to be explored on it's own to determine if they are part of the current complaint or due to another issue
- Perform a thorough systems review

- In the clinical assessment tasks, there are a large number of points associated with determining the patient's perspective but it is also useful to ask these questions in order to determine the patient's agenda
  - **Ideas**: Do you have any idea about what might be causing your symptoms?
  - **Concerns**: Is there anything in particular that has been worrying you about this?
  - **Expectations**: What were you hoping we could do for you today?
  - **Feelings and effect**: How has all of this left you feeling?

  How has this affected your life?
- To complete a thorough history, you need to include the following domains:
  - Past obstetrical/gynae/menstrual/sexual history
  - Past medical/surgical history
  - Medication history and allergies
  - Family history
  - Social history (including home life, stressors, occupation, personal habits—diet, illicit drugs, and exercise, and if appropriate travel history)

Building the relationship

- Active listening is more than just listening to what they are saying but listening for the meaning
- Ensure that your speech is slow, calm and friendly. Your tone of voice should remain consistent but adjust in relation to your patient's tone (e.g. if your patient has a low tone of voice because they are sad or upset, try to match this)
  - This technique is called mirroring which is also used to mimic the patient's body posture. Mirroring is a form of non-verbal communication that lets the patient known that you understand what they are telling you
- The patient will often express their perspective through their emotions. It is important for the purpose of exam and real life, to pick up on these cues (recognize), acknowledge them and validate these concerns ('It must be very difficult for you to continue working while you are feeling this way')
- Summarizing is also a technique that is often marked as part of process as it let's the patient know that you have been listening. It is also a helpful way of confirming the timeline of events
- Signposting prepares the patient for the next element of the consultation and makes them feel like a greater part of the team
- Empathy should be used throughout the entire consultation. This includes showing that you understand the patient's feelings and the ability to communicate this back supportively (Chafer, 2007)

Explanation and planning

The aims of information giving are to provide the patients with the appropriate amount and type of information, to deliver it in a way that ensures understanding and recall and to encourage the patient to work collaboratively in the management of their condition.

Information Type and Amount:

- Start by ascertaining the patient's starting point. Depending on the scenario, you may need to ask them how much they know about a new diagnosis or in the event of breaking bad news, you may want to ask them how much they know about the investigations that they were having

- The next element is determining how much information the patient actually wants to know. This could be form of 'I would like to tell you about what external cephalic version entails. Are you somebody who usually likes to know a lot of information or just the basics?'
- Determine if the patient has any specific questions that they would like answered
- Set the agenda taking into account your own and that of the patient Outline this to the patient and confirm that they are happy to continue

Facilitating Recall and Understanding:

- Deliver the information to the patient in a clear and unambiguous form avoiding the use of medical jargon
- Chunk the information in to manageable amounts as outlined by the initial agenda
- After each chunk, check the patient's understanding

Working Collaboratively:

- Offer the patient choices in the management of their condition. Always be aware that doing nothing is an option. Discuss the pros and cons of each.
  - A useful mnemonic to use when consenting for a procedure is DR B CAPS
    - **D**—Description
    - **R**—Risks
    - **B**—Benefits
    - **C**—Consequences of not going forward with the treatment
    - **A**—Alternative options
    - **P**—Pre-procedure and post-procedure information
    - **S**—Safeguarding
- Ask the patient if they have any concerns about what has been discussed or if they feel that there will be any obstacles

Closing the session

- Start to close the session by summarizing the most important aspects of the consultation
- Contracting is the process of agreeing to the next stage of treatment, assigning responsibility to the doctor and the patient
- Safety net by telling re-iterating to the patient what to expect going forward and warning signs that might require medical assistance
- Provide the patient with access to further information either in the form of a leaflet or giving them contact information of someone who might be able to answer further questions
- Finally close the session by checking that the patient is happy with the intended plan and then thanking them for coming to see you

Further reading

Chafer A. Communication Skills Manual. Luton & Dunstable VTS [internet]. 2003. Available from: http://www.essentialgptrainingbook.com/resources/web_chapter_04/communication%20skill%20manual%20by%20luton.pdf

Changes to the MRCOG exam in September 2016. Royal College of Obstetricians and Gynaecologists [internet]. 2016. Available from: https://www.rcog.org.uk/en/careers-training/mrcog-exams/changes-to-the-mrcog-exam-in-september-2016/

Fernando SM. Communication Skills and Counselling. *Sri Lanka Journal of Obstetrics and Gynaecology*. 2011; 33: 69–71. Kurtz SM, Silverman JD. The Calgary-Cambridge Reference Observation Guides: An aid to defining the curriculum and organizing the teaching in communication training programmes. *Medical Education*. 1996; 30: 83–9.

Neighbour R. *The Inner Consultation: how to develop an effective and intuitive consulting style*. 2nd edition. 2004. Oxford: Radcliffe Medical Press.

Skills You Need. Body Language, Posture and Proximity. [internet]. 2015. Available from: http://www.skillsyouneed.com/ips/body-language.html

Tongue JR, Epps HR, Forese LL. Communication Skills for Patient-Centered Care. *The Journal of Bone and Joint Surgery*. 2005; 87 (3).

Chapter 2 **Clinical skills**

Task 1 **Data interpretation**

Instructions for Candidate

This task assesses the following clinical skills:

- Patient safety
- Communication with patients and their relatives
- Information gathering
- Applied clinical knowledge

Mrs Zari Sardogan has a history of six weeks amenorrhoea, a positive pregnancy test and has presented with spotting PV. You are the registrar in the Early Pregnancy Assessment Unit.

Your task is:

- Take a focused history
- Interpret the data and
- Discuss management option

You have 10 minutes for this task (+ 2mins initial reading time).

Instructions for Assessor

Please read the instruction to candidate.

This clinical assessment task is to assess the skills of the candidate to take a focused history and organize appropriate investigations, reach a diagnosis and discuss the management options.

They are expected only to organize transvaginal ultrasound, *Beta* HCG and progesterone at the outset.

Show them the results of the investigations as they request them.

Results Sheet A—ask them to interpret and arrange the next test
Results Sheet B—*Beta* HCG
Results Sheet C—Progesterone

As the patient is asymptomatic, after due counselling, they should organize a repeat *beta* HCG in 48 hrs.

Results Sheet D—*Beta* HCG (48 hrs after)

As the *beta* HCG rise is suboptimal but more than 33%, the candidate may spontaneously or based on Zari's wishes organize a repeat *beta* HCG and a repeat ultrasound.

Results Sheet E—*Beta* HCG (48 hrs after Results Sheet D)
Results Sheet F—Ask them to interpret and discuss the management options

Record your overall clinical impression of the candidate for each domains (i.e. should this performance be pass, borderline, or a fail).

Here are the results:

Results Sheet A
Date xx/xx/xxxx
Zari Sardogan
Date of Birth: dd/mm/yy
Hospital no: xyx
Normal appearance of uterus, tubes and ovaries.
Endometrial thickness 12mm
No intrauterine gestational sac.
Minimal free fluid in the pelvis
Generalized probe tenderness

Results Sheet B
Date xx/xx/xxxx
Zari Sardogan
Date of Birth: dd/mm/yy
Hospital no: xyx
Beta HCG = 1400IU/ml

Results Sheet C
Date xx/xx/xxxx
Zari Sardogan
Date of Birth: dd/mm/yy
Hospital no: xyx
Progesterone = 14nmols/L

Results Sheet D
Date xx/xx/xxxx
Zari Sardogan
Date of Birth: dd/mm/yy
Hospital no: xyx
Beta HCG after 48 hrs: 2000IU/ml

Results Sheet E
Date xx/xx/xxxx
Zari Sardogan
Date of Birth: dd/mm/yy
Hospital no: xyx
Beta HCG after 48 hrs from D:
2400IU/ml

Results Sheet F (either done with result sheet E or one week after the last scan)
Date xx/xx/xxxx
Zari Sardogan
Date of Birth: dd/mm/yy
Hospital no: xyx
Fluid seen in the intrauterine cavity

No intrauterine gestational sac with triple sign noted.
2cms adnexal mass noted in the left adnexa.
Left ovary seen separate to the mass and normal. Right ovary Normal.
Minimal free fluid in the pelvis.
Probe tenderness mainly on the left.

Instruction for Role Player

You are Zari Sardogan, 36, and work as a drama teacher.

You divorced about a year ago and are currently in a relationship with RobinWarsop, 29, for the last six months.

You had been married for 14 years. You were unable to conceive and had undergone investigations for the same. You were told that you were ovulating and that your ex-husbands sperm count was normal. You were to undergo further tests to check your tubes and your GP was considering referring you for consideration for IVF. However as you are a heavy smoker, that had to be delayed. You already had a strained relationship with your ex-husband and this did not help.

You decided not to undergo any further tests.

Since the divorce, Robin is your first sexual partner. As you had not been able to conceive for so long, you had presumed that you can never become pregnant. Although you use condoms, you have had unprotected sex at least a couple of times.

So, you were surprised when you missed a period and the pregnancy test was positive.

Although Robin is not best pleased about the pregnancy, but you are secretly pleased and would be happy to carry on on your own if need be. Your last period was about six weeks ago and your periods have always been regular at 28 days.

You had some spotting this morning and a few twinges in the tummy lower down. You contacted the GP surgery and they referred you to the early pregnancy assessment unit.

You do not have any other gynaecological, surgical or medical problems. Your cervical smears have been normal and regular for the past ten years. You did have an abnormal smear requiring colposcopy and treatment ten years ago.

You smoke 20 cigarettes a day.

Temperament: You are a very emotional person and burst into tears on smallest provocation. You are known to make decisions by tour heart rather than with your head. Therefore when the candidate will tell you after the first scan and blood test that it may be early pregnancy, but with low progesterone unlikely to be viable, or there is a chance that it could be ectopic pregnancy, you will cry but not inconsolably to affect the task.

After the second blood test as the *beta* HCG has risen by 33% but not 50%, the candidate may still not be able to tell you if this is an intrauterine pregnancy, but if not spontaneously offered, you ask for one more *beta* HCG in 48 hours, as apart from the few twinges and the tenderness during the transvaginal probe, you are ok in yourself.

Ideas: You had come hoping to see a baby with a heartbeat. But you are determined to give every possible chance that it is an intrauterine pregnancy, before you agree to any treatment. You will insist on a repeat scan after the third *beta* HCG which may be organized either on the same day or a week after the first scan.

You do not want to undergo surgery and will want to consider the treatment with Methotrexate.

Concerns: You had always blamed yourself and your smoking, or so you were told, for being unable to conceive and are very concerned that you may not have an ongoing pregnancy.

Expectations: You expect the candidate to be sensitive towards you and understand where you are coming from and not insist on any treatment until you are ready.

Assessment

Marking Scheme

Patient safety:

Pass	Borderline	Fail

Communication with patients and their relatives:

Pass	Borderline	Fail

Information gathering:

Pass	Borderline	Fail

Applied clinical knowledge:

Pass	Borderline	Fail

Notes for Marking

Patient safety

- Confirms patient details and date of test
- Gives options and discusses the pros and cons
- Aware of the limitations of ultrasound
- Counsels the patient to report if pain or feels unwell while awaiting the repeat *beta* HCG-s
- Honest
- Does not try to give blanket answers when unsure

Communication with patient

- Clear and concise communication with the assessor
- Greets, appropriate introduction
- Creates rapport with the patient
- Sensitive to patient's needs.
- Explains agenda of the meeting and checks her agenda
- Determine her existing understandings and explores her concerns
- Clear organized explanation in logical sequence chunks: language avoids medical jargon
- Provides information leaflets
- Demonstrates reliable counselling skills

Information gathering

- Obtains a focussed and relevant gynaecological, sexua,l and social history
- Obtains views, expectations, and concerns
- Able to understand the patient's point of view

Applied clinical knowledge

- Aware uterus may be seen empty under *beta* HCG—1500iu
- Free fluid in the pelvis may indicate bleeding
- Realizes the importance of probe tenderness may be indicative of ectopic pregnancy
- Above 1500iu intrauterine pregnancy seen on transvaginal scan
- Aware that this progesterone level unlikely to be suggestive of an early viable pregnancy
- *Beta* HCG doubles in 48hour with intrauterine ongoing pregnancy
- Suboptimal (less than double) in ectopic pregnancy or failing pregnancy
- Discusses the need for a third *Beta* HCG to confirm diagnosis
- Discusses treatment options (medical (Methotrexate) vs surgical) including the pros and cons
- Discusses other blood tests needed before Methotrexate
- Aware of risk of recurrence of ectopic pregnancy and recommends an early scan in the next pregnancy

Further reading

Elson CJ, Salim R, Potdar N, Chetty M, Ross JA, Kirk EJ on behalf of the Royal College of Obstetricians and Gynaecologists. Diagnosis and management of ectop ic pregnancy. BJOG 2016;.123:e15–e55.

Diagnosis and Management of Ectopic Pregnancy (Green-top Guideline No. 21; Joint with the Association of Early Pregnancy Units) 04/11/2016 https://www.rcog.org.uk/en/guidelines-research-services/guidelines/gtg21/

Ectopic pregnancy and miscarriage: diagnosis and initial management, Clinical guideline[CG154 Published date: December 2012 https://www.nice.org.uk/guidance/cg154

Task 2 **Clinical reasoning**

Instructions for Candidate

This task assesses the following clinical skills:

- Patient safety
- Communication with patients and their relatives
- Information gathering
- Applied clinical knowledge

You have 10 minutes for this task (+ 2mins initial reading time).

Freya King is a 38-year-old lady in her first pregnancy. She has no other health problems and her pregnancy has progressed well so far.

She is currently 41 weeks pregnant and has been referred by her community midwife to the antenatal clinic to discuss further management regarding her pregnancy and delivery.

Your task is to:

- discuss the management options
- come to an agreement with the patient regarding the next stage in the management

Instructions for Assessor

Please read the instruction to the candidate.

This Clinical assessment task is to assess the candidate's ability to take a focussed history and counsel the patient regarding the options for management of post- pregnancy dates. They should be able to conveys the pros, cons, and risks and counsel the patient in a non-judgemental way. Although, they should be clear in conveying the risks of continuing pregnancy after 42 weeks, they should respect the patient's decision and organize the necessary surveillance. Record your overall clinical impression of the candidate for each domains (i.e. should this performance be pass, borderline, or a fail).

Instruction for Role Player

You are Freya King, a 38year-old florist.

You are healthy and so far your pregnancy had progressed smoothly and you feel good baby movements. The Downs syndrome screening test, blood tests and the baby's scan at 20 weeks have all been normal.

You had been given a due date of one week ago, but so far you have had no signs of going into labour.

One of your friends underwent induction of labour at the hospital as she was overdue. This was complicated. She had to wait until a bed was available on the delivery floor to break the waters after the tablets. She then needed an emergency caesarean and lost about four litres of blood requiring blood transfusion. She has found the whole episode very traumatic and has found it very difficult to bond with the baby.

You believe in the power of nature and hate hospitals. You were planning a home birth and the only times you have come to the hospital; were for your scans.

You have no medical problems or allergies.

Temperament: You are a very calm person but also quite adamant. You are not confrontational but stick to your ground in a calm fashion.

Ideas: You want to wait until nature takes its course. Your baby is moving well, so you intend to carry on beyond 42 weeks if required. You do not want to be induced. You want a nice calm home delivery. But if the candidate is respecting your decision and convinces you to have a hospital delivery, you may agree.

Concerns: You are concerned that the doctor (candidate) may make you feel guilty by scaring you about the possibility of harm to your baby if you wait longer than 42 weeks and try to coerce you to undergo an induction.

Expectations: You want to have a non-judgemental discussion. You want to know what to report if you wait beyond 42 weeks and what can the doctor put in place to help you carry on.

You are happy to listen to the option of induction but have already made up your mind not to undergo the induction.

Assessment

Marking Scheme

Patient safety:

Pass Borderline Fail

Communication with patients and their relatives:

Pass Borderline Fail

Information gathering:

Pass Borderline Fail

Applied clinical knowledge:

Pass Borderline Fail

Notes for Marking

Patient safety

- Counsels the fetus and maternal risks of continuing pregnancy after 42 weeks and not recommended
- Puts in place foetal surveillance by alternate day twice weekly CTG and weekly ultrasound for amniotic fluid
- Advises to monitor baby movements and report if concerns
- Advises to deliver in the hospital. if delivery after 42 weeks in view of increased foetal risks including meconium aspiration

Communication with patient

- Non-judgemental
- Clear and concise communication with the assessor
- Greets, appropriate introduction
- Creates rapport with the patient
- Sensitive to patients needs
- Explains agenda of the meeting and checks her agenda
- Determine her existing understandings and explores her concerns
- Clear organized explanation in logical sequence chunks: language avoids medical jargon

- Provides information leaflets
- Demonstrates reliable counselling skills

Information gathering

- Obtains a relevant obstetric history
- Obtains views, expectations, and concerns regarding induction, labou,r and delivery

Applied clinical knowledge

- Post-term pregnancy (more than 42 weeks) is associated with an increase in perinatal morbidity and otherwise unexplained perinatal mortality in structurally normal babies
- The perinatal mortality rate, defined as stillbirths plus early neonatal deaths, at 42 weeks of gestation is twice as high as that at term (4–7 vs 2–3 per 1000 deliveries, respectively). It increases 4-fold at 43 weeks and 5–7-fold at 44 weeks
- Foetal morbidity is also increased in postterm pregnancies and pregnancies that progress beyond 41 weeks gestation. This includes passage of meconium, meconium aspiration syndrome, macrosomia and dysmaturity. Post term pregnancy also is an independent risk factor for low umbilical cord pH levels (neonatal acidaemia), low 5-minute Apgar scores
- Postterm pregnancy is associated with significant risks to the mother. There is an increased risk of: 1) labour dystocia (9–12% vs 2–7% at term); 2) severe perineal lacerations (3rd and 4th degree tears), related to macrosomia (3.3% vs 2.6% at term); 3) operative vaginal delivery; and 4) doubling in caesarean section (CS) rates (14% vs 7% at term
- Options:
  - Membrane sweep
  - Induction of labour between term + 10 to term + 14 days
  - Expectant management—recommended up to 42 weeks

Further reading

Inducing labour, Nice Clinical guideline [CG70] Published date: July 2008. https://www.nice.org.uk/guidance/cg70

Hilder L, Costeloe K, Thilaganathan B. Prolonged pregnancy: evaluating gestation-specific risks of fetal and infant mortality. *British Journal of Obstetrics & Gynaecology*. 1998; 105: 169–73.

Cotzias CS, Brown S, Fisk NM. Prospective risk of unexplained stillbirth in singleton pregnancies at term: population based analysis. *British Medical Journal*. 1999; 319: 287–8.

Treger M, Hallak M, Silberstein T, et al. Post-term pregnancy: should induction of labor be considered before 42 weeks? *The Journal of Maternal-Fetal & Neonatal Medicine*. 2002;11: 50–53.

M. Galal, I. Symonds, H. Murray, F. Petraglia, and R. Smith Postterm pregnancy, *Facts Views & Visions in Obstetrics & Gynaecology*. 2012; 4(3): 175–87.

Chapter 3 **Teaching appraisal and assessment**

Task 1 **Teaching skills**

Instructions for Candidate

This task assesses the following clinical skills:

- Patient Safety
- Communication with colleagues
- Applied clinical knowledge

You are teaching practical management of shoulder dystocia to your ST1 doctor who has just started obstetrics. He/she has witnessed a shoulder dystocia after a forceps delivery last week and is very stressed about facing one.

You have a pelvis and baby model and today you are teaching the shoulder dystocia scenario.

You have 10 minutes for this task (+ 2mins initial reading time).

Instructions for Assessor

This station assesses the candidate's ability to teach a practical skill. This will also assess their knowledge of managing shoulder dystocia.

Please observe the teaching and do not interrupt.

Instructions for Role Player

You are a ST1 doctor who has just completed the foundation training. This is your second week on the delivery suite. You have seen one shoulder dystocia after forceps delivery recently. You found the experience stressful and are now worried about facing such a scenario. Your Registrar has kindly agreed to teach you the practical management of Shoulder dystocia using the pelvis and baby model.

Please do not prompt and follow the instructions of the candidate (registrar).

Assessment

Marking Scheme

Patient safety:

Pass	Borderline	Fail

Communication with colleagues:

Pass	Borderline	Fail

Applied clinical knowledge:

Pass	Borderline	Fail

Notes for Marking

Patient safety

- Avoid dangerous manoeuvres fundal pressure and excessive lateral and downward traction
- Explain advanced techniques and advice the importance of using them only if experienced—Zavanelli's manoeuvre and symphysiotomy
- Explains the importance of documentation

Communication with colleagues

- Explains the objectives of the station
- Allows active involvement of the team/trainee
- Promotes team working
- Makes the trainee demonstrate while talking through the steps and allows trainee to talk through while demonstrating
- Finally gives opportunity to the trainee to independently talk through and demonstrate the whole scenario

Applied clinical knowledge

- Has knowledge of all the manoeuvres
- Demonstrates and talks through the steps
- Recognize the problem
- Call for help
- Mc Roberts manoeuvre
- Suprapubic pressure
- Consider episiotomy
- Posterior arm delivery or internal rotatory manoeuvres
- Turn into all fours
- Emphasize subsequent management
- If unsuccessful consider repeating the manoeuvres
- If experienced, consider advanced manoeuvres
- Complete delivery. Explains to anticipate post delivery problems (PPH, neonatal resuscitation, genital tract trauma)
- Check paired cord gases

Further reading

RCOG: Shoulder Dystocia (Green-top Guideline No. 42. https://www.rcog.org.uk/en/guidelines-research-services/guidelines/gtg42/

Task 2 **Teaching instrumental delivery**

Instructions for Candidate

This task assesses the following clinical skills:

- Patient Safety
- Communication with colleagues
- Applied clinical knowledge

You have a new FY2 who has requested an informal teaching on operative vaginal delivery, particularly forceps delivery. The trainee will have some questions around the following points:

- Pre-requisites of operative vaginal delivery
- Application of the instrument
- Amount and direction of traction
- Choice of instrument

You are not expected to talk about indications of instrumental delivery or anything else outside the above mentioned points. The examiner will act as the junior doctor and will ask you questions through the discussion revolving around the above mentioned points.

You have 10 minutes for this task. (+ 2mins initial reading time).

Instructions for Assessor

This is a teaching station and the candidate should demonstrate their understanding of:

- the principles of adult learning
- the skills and practices of a competent teacher
- the principles of giving feedback
- the principles of evaluation
- Teaching strategies appropriate to adult learning

These skills should be demonstrated by balancing the needs of service delivery with education. Use the criteria mentioned below in the marking scheme to ensure an up-to mark teaching session.

Instructions for Role Player

You are a second year foundation year doctor just starting your career in obstetrics and gynaecology. You are quite enthusiastic and keen on learning things in the right way.

You are already aware of the indications of instrumental delivery and do not want to waste time in that repetition. You have gone through the RCOG Green-top guideline on operative vaginal delivery. You are more interested to know the handling of the instrument and the procedure steps. Your concern is that you don't want to start doing the procedure unless you have discussed it thoroughly with a senior, while you also acknowledge your senior is busy.

The candidate must appreciate your enthusiasm and reciprocate it by showing willingness to answer all your questions and identifying your learning needs.

You expect to be taught around the following points:

- Pre-requisites of operative vaginal delivery
- Application of the instrument

- Amount and direction of traction
- Choice of instrument

You can ask additional questions during the teaching session when invited by the candidate.

- When can we not perform an operative delivery? (The candidate should talk about the pre-requisites of operative delivery as mentioned in Green-top guideline)
- How to apply the forceps? How to ensure that the instrument is applied safely?
- How much force can you use for the pull? Is there a specific direction for the pull?
- What makes you decide between a vacuum extraction and a forceps delivery?(Clinical circumstances, operators skills, availability of equipment)
- Can I apply a ventouse if the application of forceps fails for some reason?
- How can I gain proficiency in instrumental delivery? (attending skills and drills and using OSATS)
- How many instrument deliveries should I perform under supervision before performing unsupervized? (No data exists of number of supervized procedures necessary before gaining proficiency. Should be decided between a specified trainer and the trainee)

Assessment

Marking scheme

Patient safety:

Pass	Borderline	Fail

Communication with colleagues:

Pass	Borderline	Fail

Applied clinical knowledge:

Pass	Borderline	Fail

Notes for Marking

Patient safety

The candidate must include following points of safety and quality:

- Demonstrates ability to identify risk factors
- When to involve a consultant
- Demonstrates understanding of clinical governance and risk management
- Suggest adequate training in the form of skills and drills
- Highlights importance of adherence to policies and procedures

Communication with colleagues

- Demonstrates ability to teach appropriate skills to other colleagues in a logical and coherent manner with recognition of the learner, environment and resources available
- Establishes the learning needs
- Check pre-existing knowledge
- Use the resources provided
- Uses a variety of teaching methods e.g. illustrations, models, etc.
- Checks information intake, needs met

- Two-way feedback
- Offer reading references

Applied clinical Knowledge

- The candidate should be able to demonstrate honesty where there is clinical uncertainty on examination findings and appropriateness of the procedure. They should demonstrate their ability to emphasize on importance of clinical examination findings in the context of the clinical scenario and choice of instrument. They should be able to demonstrate awareness of the risks and benefits of both options balancing needs of mother and foetus (ventouse and forceps)

Notes for Candidate

The scenario is about one of the most common obstetric procedures. It not only assesses the process of communication as a teacher but also assesses the content of the knowledge around the subject. It is important how you deliver the information in a teaching session.

Practice this scenario with one of your friends who can act as a role player and ask another friend to provide you with feedback.

Further reading

Green–top Guideline No. 26, Operative Vaginal Delivery, Royal College of Obstetricians and Gynaecologists. https://www.rcog.org.uk/globalassets/documents/guidelines/gtg_26.pdf

Sinha P, Dutta A, and Langford A. Instrumental delivery: how to meet the need for improvements in training. *The Obstetrician & Gynaecologist*, 2010; 12(4): 265–71.

Chapter 4 **Information technology, clinical governance, and research**

Task 1 **Audit**

Instructions for Candidate

This task assesses the following clinical skills:

Patient safety
Communication with colleagues
Applied clinical knowledge

In Box 4.1 are the findings of an audit on Service provision of Termination of Pregnancy.

Your task is to:

- Go through the findings in the first six minutes
- In the next six minutes you will be asked to critically appraise the methodology and results of the audit

You have 12 minutes for this task. Use the 2 minute initial reading time to start going through the article findings.

Instructions for Assessor

The candidate has six minutes to prepare for this station. Please do not interrupt them in this time.

Ask them to critically appraise the audit. If you need to prompt, adjust the marks accordingly.

You may need to prompt them to comment on why the audit was done, the appropriateness and limitations of the methodology, findings, and the implications for change in practice.

Assessment

Marking Scheme

Patient safety:

Pass	Borderline	Fail

Communication with patients and their relatives:

Pass	Borderline	Fail

Information gathering:

Pass	Borderline	Fail

Applied clinical knowledge:

Pass	Borderline	Fail

Box 4.1 Findings of an audit on Service provision of Termination of Pregnancy

- 55 women, 24.02.15–01.09.15
- Two continued pregnancies, one miscarriage
- National standards from RCOG Care of women requesting abortion
- 48MTOP, 4STOP
- TOP <24/40 -100%
- Written, objective, evidence-guided information is available for women considering abortion to take away before the procedure—100%
- Women who decide to continue with the pregnancy should be referred for antenatal care without delay—2/55—letter to GP
- Women who have a non-viable pregnancy require appropriate management—1/55—surgical management
- 2 signatures from doctors on HSA1 form—50/52, 2 forms missing, DATIX completed and investigated
- Consent form signed, explanation of risks—procedure-specific consent form—100%
- Blood tests—100%
- Chlamydia screening offered—100%
- Antibiotic prophylaxis—1/52 not documented whether antibiotics were given
- Anti-D prophylaxis—one woman declined despite explanation
- All women undergoing an abortion should undergo a venous thromboembolism (VTE) risk assessment—none
- All appropriate methods of contraception should be discussed with women at the initial assessment and a plan agreed for contraception after the abortion—100%
- Documented evidence of contraceptive advice—96%
- All women undergoing an abortion should undergo a venous thromboembolism (VTE) risk assessment—none
- DoH notification (Yellow form)—100%
- Recommendations—the original Certificate A will never leave the patient notes. Any usage of the certificate A will be with a copy of the certificate clearly marked as COPY
- TRA form to be filled though the drug chart is used on the proforma.
- Staff reminded of importance of documentation of antibiotics given and contraception advice discussion
- Re-audit in six months

Notes for Marking

Patient safety

- Are any of the practices harmful/affecting adversely the patient's safety? Has this been recognized and changes made before the completion of audit?
- Is patient service user included in the audit? (Type a quote from the document or the summary of an interesting point. You can position the text box anywhere in the document.)
- Is it a patient survey questionnaire?
- Is the confidentiality maintained

Communication with colleague

- Explains why a particular topic was chosen
- Explains which national/local standards are chosen
- Explains if data is collected appropriately
- Explains where the results were discussed
- Explains if any robust plans for re-audit are in place
- Explains if re-audit results are presented in this presentation

Applied clinical knowledge

- Understands what a clinical audit is and the cycle.
- Understands what an audit is not about
- Understands the difference between audit and research
- Selecting a topic—service evaluation
- Standards of best practice (audit criteria).
- Collecting data—time frame, notes collection method, any omissions
- Analysing data against standards—-National/local guidelines
- Feeding back results—where results discussed, how results are disseminated
- Discussing possible changes—identifying the problem areas and action plan
- Implementing agreed changes—how? Resources? Staffing?
- Allowing time for changes to embed before re-auditing—plan for re-audit? When?
- Collecting a second set of data—is the cycle completed?
- Analysing the re-audit data—understands to compare against the same audit criteria, no change in guidelines since previous audit?
- Feeding back the re-audit results
- Discussing whether practice has improved

Further reading

StratOG: https://stratog.rcog.org.uk/tutorial/clinical-audit

RCOG Clinical Governance Advice, No. 5 https://www.rcog.org.uk/globalassets/documents/guidelines/clinical-governance-advice/clingov5understandingaudit2003.pdf

Task 2 **Risk management**

Instructions for Candidate

This task assesses the following clinical skills:

- Patient safety
- Communication with colleagues
- Applied clinical knowledge

It has been brought to your attention that some of the results of genital swabs performed for emergency patients on gynaecology ward have not been checked in the last three months.

A 19-year-old girl had been reviewed three months ago on the Emergency Gynaecology ward for lower abdominal pain. Clinical examination had shown normal vitals, soft abdomen with minimal tenderness in the left iliac fossa and no signs of peritonism.

Her pregnancy test was negative; bloods were normal, urine dipstick negative. Genital swabs were taken and sent to microbiology.

An urgent ultrasound scan was organized and showed no abnormalities. She was reassured, advised to take regular laxatives and discharged with no further follow up.

Her Chlamydia swab was reported as positive. However, no action has been taken for the last three months.

Now you have to discuss the next steps with the risk manager.

You have 10 minutes for this station (+ 2 minutes of initial reading time).

Instructions for Assessor

This task assesses the candidate's ability to communicate an incident and discuss the implications of the incident. They are supposed to suggest recommendations to prevent a recurrence of such an event.

You will also role play as the risk manager. If you need to prompt, adjust the scoring accordingly.

You may need to ask them:

Risk identification—what went wrong?

Risk analysis and evaluation—what are the chances of it going wrong and what would be the impact?

Risk treatment—what can we do to minimize the chance of this happening?

Assessment

Marking Scheme

Patient safety:

Pass	Borderline	Fail

Communication with patients and their relatives:

Pass	Borderline	Fail

Applied clinical knowledge:

Pass	Borderline	Fail

Notes for Marking

Patient safety

- Risk identification—what went wrong?—What are the systems in place for checking the test results for emergency admissions? Why this has been missed?
- Risk analysis and evaluation—what are the chances of it going wrong and what would be the impact?—any other important investigation for other patients missed? Any untoward consequences due to missed results?
- Risk treatment—what can we do to minimize the chance of this happening or to mitigate damage when it has gone wrong?—Robust systems in place for checking results, named responsibility, escalation.
- Risk control sharing and learning—what can we learn from things that have gone wrong?—Incident form filling, audit of all emergency admissions, discussion at clinical governance meeting, and dissemination of results to all junior and senior medical staff
- Duty of Candour—open to the patient regarding delay in treatment due to missed result, impact of delay in treatment, follow up

Communication with colleagues

- Presents the detailed history and timeline with facts to the risk manager
- Avoids personal opinion and gives unbiased report

Applied clinical knowledge

- Implications of delay in the treatment
- Treatment
- Contact tracing
- Test of cure
- GUM screening

Further reading

StratOG: https://stratog.rcog.org.uk/tutorial/clinical-governance/risk-management-279
RCOG: Improving Patient Safety: Risk Management for Maternity and Gynaecology (Clinical Governance Advice No. 2) https://www.rcog.org.uk/en/guidelines-research-services/guidelines/clinical-governance-advice-2/

Task 3 **Research methodology and statistics**

Instructions for Candidate

This task assesses the following clinical skills:

- Patient safety
- Communication with colleagues
- Applied clinical knowledge

In Box 4.2 is an abstract of the OPPTIMUM trial published in the Lancet, February 2016. Your task is to:

- Go through the findings in the first seven minutes
- In the next five minutes you will be asked to critically appraise the study

You have 12 minutes for this task. Use the two minute initial reading time to start going through the article findings.

Instructions to Assessor

The candidates had 7 minutes to prepare for this station. Please do not disturb them during this time/ Ask them to critically appraise the study. If you need to prompt, adjust the marks accordingly. You may need to prompt them to comment on the

- What was the main research question behind this study?
- What is the study?
- What are the strengths and weaknesses of the study?
- What are the main conclusions of the study and how do you think they should affect current practice?

Assessment

Marking Scheme

Patient safety:

Pass Borderline Fail

Communication with patients and their relatives:

Pass Borderline Fail

Applied clinical knowledge:

Pass Borderline Fail

Notes for Marking

Patient safety

- Addresses an important obstetric problem
- Check ethical approval
- Check safety outcomes, adverse events addressed
- Unbiased explanation

Box 4.2 Abstract of the OPPTIMUM trial

Background

Progesterone administration has been shown to reduce the risk of preterm birth and neonatal morbidity in women at high risk, but there is uncertainty about longer term effects on the child.

Methods

We did a double-blind, randomized, multicentric, placebo-controlled trial of vaginal progesterone, 200mg daily taken from 22–24 to 34 weeks of gestation, on pregnancy and infant outcomes in women at risk of preterm birth (because of previous spontaneous birth at ≤34 weeks and 0 days of gestation, or a cervical length ≤25 mm, or because of a positive foetal fibronectin test combined with other clinical risk factors for preterm birth [any one of a history in a previous pregnancy of preterm birth, second trimester loss, preterm premature foetal membrane rupture, or a history of a cervical procedure to treat abnormal smears]). The objective of the study was to determine whether vaginal progesterone prophylaxis given to reduce the risk of preterm birth affects neonatal and childhood outcomes. We defined three primary outcomes: foetal death or birth before 34 weeks and 0 days gestation (obstetric), a composite of death, brain injury, or bronchopulmonary dysplasia (neonatal), and a standardized cognitive score at two years of age (childhood), imputing values for deaths. Randomization was done through a web portal, with participants, investigators, and others involved in giving the intervention, assessing outcomes, or analysing data masked to treatment allocation until the end of the study. Analysis was by intention to treat.

Statistical Analysis

A statistical analysis plan was finalized before data lock. Statistical analyses were done by C-MM and AM at the Robertson Centre for Biostatistics, Glasgow University according to the intention-to-treat principle. The three primary outcomes and secondary outcomes were compared between the treatment groups using mixed effects logistic regression (or, for continuous variables, linear regression) models including treatment allocation and previous pregnancy (≥14 weeks) as fixed effects, with study centre as a random effect. According to the pre-specified statistical analysis plan, p values were initially reported without adjustment for multiple comparisons, and then adjusted using a Bonferroni-Holm procedure. The planned sample size was around 1125 participants, depending on the relative numbers of foetal fibronectin-positive and foetal fibronectin-negative women recruited. Detailed sample size calculations are available in the published protocol, but in brief the study had at least 80% power to detect what was considered the minimal important clinical difference for each of the three primary outcomes at a nominal 5% level of significance.

Sensitivity analyses included repeating the primary analyses in a per-protocol dataset (which excluded data from women who were found not to be compliant with the inclusion or exclusion criteria, or who had a structural or chromosomal foetal anomaly discovered after inclusion, or who had a multiple pregnancy discovered after inclusion or who were not adequately compliant with treatment by the pre-specified definition), and the use of multiple imputation of missing primary outcome data. Preplanned subgroup analyses for primary outcomes were done by extending the main regression models to include interaction terms for the following subgroups: fibronectin positive or fibronectin negative, cervical length of at most 25mm or longer than 25mm, cervical length of at most 15mm or longer than 15mm, chorioamnionitis yes or no, history of spontaneous preterm birth or no such history, and history of preterm birth or no such history. Safety outcomes (adverse events) were assessed in a safety population, excluding women for whom it was documented that no study medication was taken.

Findings

Between 2 Feb 2009, and 12 April 2013, we randomly assigned 1228 women to the placebo group (n = 610) and the progesterone group (n = 618). In the placebo group, data from 597, 587, and

(*continued*)

Box 4.2 *Continued*

439 women or babies were available for analysis of obstetric, neonatal, and childhood outcomes, respectively; in the progesterone group the corresponding numbers were 600, 589, and 430. After correction for multiple outcomes, progesterone had no significant effect on the primary obstetric outcome (odds ratio adjusted for multiple comparisons [OR] 0·86, 95% CI 0·61–1·22) or neonatal outcome (OR 0·62, 0·38–1·03), nor on the childhood outcome (cognitive score, progesterone group vs placebo group, 97·3 [SD 17·9] vs 97·7 [17·5]; difference in means −0·48, 95% CI −2·77 to 1·81). Maternal or child serious adverse events were reported in 70 (11%) of 610 patients in the placebo group and 59 (10%) of 616 patients in the progesterone group (p = 0·27).

Interpretation

Vaginal progesterone was not associated with reduced risk of preterm birth or composite neonatal adverse outcomes, and had no long-term benefit or harm on outcomes in children at two years of age

Communication with colleague

- Explain whether a good study
- Explains Positives and negatives of the study

Applied clinical knowledge

- How to critically appraise a paper
- Study design
  - Randomized
  - Double blind
  - Multicentric
  - Placebo-controlled
- Concealed allocation
- End points are explicitly stated
- Power calculation performed
- The groups treated equally apart from experimental intervention
- Statistical methods clearly mentioned
- Intention to treat analysis
- Follow up complete

Further reading

Fowkes, FG, Critical appraisal of published research: introductory guidelines, *BMJ* 1991; 302 doi: http://dx.doi.org/10.1136/bmj.302.6785.1136 (Published 11 May 1991)

Norman, J.E, Marlow N. and Messow C et al., Vaginal progesterone prophylaxis for preterm birth (the OPPTIMUM study): a multicentre, randomised, double-blind trial, *The Lancet*, 2016; http://www.thelancet.com/journals/lancet/article/PIIS0140-6736(16)00350-0/abstract

StartOG, https://stratog.rcog.org.uk/tutorial/research/critical-appraisal-of-articles-5867

Chapter 5 **Ethical and legal issues**

Task 1 **Consent**

Instructions for Candidate

This task assesses the following clinical skills:

- Patient safety
- Communication with patients
- Information gathering
- Applied clinical knowledge

You are working alongside your consultant in the termination of pregnancy clinic and have just seen 15-year-old Chantelle Briar who has come with her friend requesting a termination of pregnancy. She insists she has a surgical termination of pregnancy as she does not want to have any pain during the procedure. Please take the appropriate consent for the procedure.

You have 10 minutes for this task. (+ 2mins initial reading time).

Instructions for Assessor

This station assesses the candidate's ability to consent and their understanding of the important principles of Gillick/Fraser competence and the issues surrounding Jehovah's witness.

Please do not interrupt them.

Instructions for Role Player

You are Chantelle Briar, 15-year-old and attending the clinic requesting termination of pregnancy. You are in the High school and are preparing for your GCSEs. You like the school and have good friends. You are training for competitive swimming and have lot of plans for your future career. You have recently been going out with one of your classmates who recently moved to your school. You have used condoms during sex but do not understand how you got pregnant. Your friend suggested you take a pregnancy test after you felt sick in your last swimming lesson and it was positive. You are shocked and worried as your parents are not aware that you are sexually active. You have not informed any of your family members or teachers or GP regarding the pregnancy. You googled for the termination services and got an appointment at the clinic. Your boyfriend is aware and is supportive; he has not informed his parents either. You wish to have surgical termination so that it is all done quickly and with no pain. Your friend has accompanied you to the clinic and has been very supportive throughout. When you are seen by the doctor you insist that it is all kept confidential and that you would not wish either your parents or your family doctor know about it. You would want the procedure to be done as soon as possible and the first thing in the morning so you could go home by the end of the day. Your friend has kindly agreed to accompany you home. You are fit and well. You are a Jehovah's witness and would not accept blood transfusion and would give this information when the doctor explains the need for blood transfusion when there is heavy bleeding during the procedure. You are happy to go to the chemists to get some contraceptive pills for future but wouldn't want the GP to prescribe it. You understand the risks and happy to sign the consent form.

Assessment

Marking Scheme

Patient safety:

Pass	Borderline	Fail

Communication with patient:

Pass	Borderline	Fail

Information gathering:

Pass	Borderline	Fail

Applied clinical knowledge:

Pass	Borderline	Fail

Notes for Marking

Patient safety

- Ensure consensual sex and no safeguarding required

Communication with patient

- Explain proposed procedure, what it involves, benefits, serious and frequently occurring risks, benefits and risks of alternative treatments, extra procedures including laparoscopy, laparotomy, repair of organ injury, anaesthesia used.
- Serious risks include:
  - Uterine perforation, up to five in 1000 women (uncommon)
  - Significant trauma to the cervix (rare)
  - There is no substantiated evidence in the literature of any impact on future fertility.

Frequent risks include:

  - Bleeding that lasts for up to 2 weeks is very common but blood transfusion is uncommon (1–2 in 1000 women)
  - Need for repeat surgical evacuation, up to five in 100 women (common)
  - Localized pelvic infection, three in 100 women (common).
- Give information leaflets
- Risk of blood transfusion, alternatives in Jehovah's witness.
- Advice regarding future contraception

Information gathering

- Obtains a focused and relevant sexual history
- Obtains a relevant history including the fact that patient is a Jehova's witness

Applied clinical knowledge

- Understand Gillick/Fraser competence
- Young women under 16 years of age are able to give their consent to undergo medical or surgical termination of pregnancy provided that they are considered to have capacity. For this age group it is advisable but not essential to involve a parent or responsible adult. It is also important to note that the putative father of a foetus cannot override or withhold consent for abortion

- Aware of advanced directives for Jehovah's witness, alternatives to blood in Jehovah's witness
- Contraception in adolescents—benefits and risks

Notes to Candidates

Be familiar with your local hospital guidelines and policies advanced directive) concerning Jehovah's witness and blood transfusion.

Further reading

RCOG: Obtaining Valid Consent (Clinical Governance Advice No. 6), https://www.rcog.org.uk/en/guidelines-research-services/guidelines/clinical-governance-advice-6/

A child's legal rights: Gillick competency and Fraser guidelines, https://www.nspcc.org.uk/preventing-abuse/child-protection-system/legal-definition-child-rights-law/gillick-competency-fraser-guidelines/

Task 2 **Legal framework for practice**

Instructions for Candidate

This task assesses the following clinical skills:

- Patient safety
- Communication with patients
- Information gathering
- Applied clinical knowledge

You are in the pre-op gynaecology clinic and have been asked to see Ellie Pryor to explain the procedure planned for her.

She is 24 years of age with severe cyclical pelvic pain in the luteal phase with dyspareunia and pain on bowel opening. Her periods are not heavy and are perfectly regular. She has never been pregnant, never had a cervical smear and has no significant medical history and no previous surgery. She is taking painkillers, smokes five cigarettes per day and drinks two to three units most nights after work. She does not have a regular partner and uses barrier methods of contraception and has no plans for children. Her body mass index is 20.

Pelvic ultrasound and MRI scans have confirmed the presence of a 6cm left sided endometrioma and no other signs of endometriosis. Examination in GOPD by her consultant has confirmed the presence of a left sided tender mass. No endometriotic nodules were seen or palpated.

In clinic, pending MRI scan, the consultant explained that Ellie would need diagnostic laparoscopy with or without treatment to endometriosis. The specialist nurse has also spoken to Ellie since the MRI and told her that she may need an ovarian cystectomy. The consultant also explained there may also be some residual disease which requires medical treatment afterwards or she may need more major surgery at a later date.

Your task is to explain the procedure planned, discuss the risks of the procedure and come to a clear agreement with the patient as to her expectations from the operation and how her management may evolve in the future.

You are not expected to complete a consent form.

You have 10 minutes for this task (+ 2mins initial reading time).

Instructions for Assessor

This station is designed to test the student's ability to manage a demanding patient in a situation where there is a need to match the expectations of appropriate clinical management with those of a patient who is prepared to do whatever it takes to sort out her problems. This is especially relevant when the patient is giving serious consideration to losing her fertility at a young age.

Allow the actor to put mild pressure on the candidate to ask for a pelvic clearance but ensure that if the candidate does not explore the middle ground of unilateral oophorectomy to reduce the risk of recurrence that the actor is seen to back down a little to ask about whether there is a middle ground.

Essentials of this case are appropriate explanation of the risks and not agreeing to a hysterectomy or bilateral oophorectomy. An excellent pass would be explaining the risks fully whilst reassuring and settling this patient with the outcome that a left salpingo-oophorectomy would be the largest procedure performed but that if the disease is so severe it may just be diagnostic with planning a larger procedure at a later date.

Instructions for Role Player

Ellie Pryor is a 24-year-old woman who has a strong suspicion of endometriosis from tests performed so far. A recent scan suggests you have a cyst in your left ovary that contains endometriosis.

You have a good understanding of the condition itself and whilst you are concerned about its existence you really just want to get rid of the pain you are getting every month. The pain is mainly on the left side, starts roughly mid cycle every month as a nagging pain and increases steadily to a crescendo just before your period and results in you having to take at least one day off work per month. In the week before your period you experience intense pain on passing a motion and are unable to have sex due to the pain. You consider your quality of life to be massively impaired by these symptoms.

You work as a sales executive in a local BMW car dealership and are currently the top performing executive with a very high chance of a large bonus and promotion to team leader. It's a cutthroat environment and nobody shows weakness. This pain infuriates you, you are not worried about the long term, you just want anything that could cause pain to be gone so that you can work and be seen to work. You are quite prepared to have everything removed to get your life back. Whilst you don't really understand the consequences of removing everything you are widely read that hysterectomy will cure your pain.

You don't want to take any drugs; your GP has tried loads already ('every type of contraception in the book'). In fact, with your documented lack of response to drugs so far you are likely to say that you are being fobbed off if anyone offers you drug therapy

You have never been pregnant, never had a cervical smear and are otherwise in excellent health with no significant medical history and no previous surgery. Apart from painkillers you take no drugs. Whilst you are an exercise addict (mainly running) you smoke five cigarettes per day and drink two to three units most nights after work with 'the lads from work'. You do not have a regular partner and use barrier methods of contraception. You have no plans for children in your life. You have an aggressive demeanor that is easily subdued in the presence of a suitably reassuring professional yet you freely admit not suffering fools gladly. Your body mass index is 20.

You went to see your GP about the problem and she was very sympathetic but said that you needed to see a gynaecologist. The gynaecologist you saw first you liked very much even though you found examination very painful. She was very thorough, requested an MRI scan and explained that you would need a diagnostic laparoscopy to explore what is going on and to plan any surgery. You have spoken to the specialist nurse who explained that the MRI is suggestive of endometriosis. She also suggested that whilst some treatment is likely to happen at the time of the laparoscopy there may also be some residual disease which requires medical treatment afterwards or you may need more major surgery.

Your aim at this pre-op consent clinic is to make sure that something definitive is done at the operation rather than just explorative. Given that the ovarian cyst is large you would rather it was removed completely as a bare minimum. Your optimal management solution would be to have a pelvic clearance with hysterectomy and removal of both ovaries as this is what happened to your mother when she was 38 after years of suffering. You have read that removal of both ovaries would prevent it coming back and that seems like a sensible solution that should be explored.

Be prepared to get emotional and cross/irritated if the candidate doesn't allow you to explore all the options and just wants to go down one route. As long as the candidate makes sense then settle for the removal of the affected ovary. Be really cross if they insist on just doing a diagnostic laparoscopy but acquiesce if they are insistent that hysterectomy and removal of ovaries is not the right thing to do now.

You will also have to accept if they say it might not be possible to entirely remove the affected ovary if at laparoscopy other high risk features/major surgery might be needed at a later date.

Assessment

Marking Scheme		
Patient safety:		
Pass	Borderline	Fail
Communication with patient:		
Pass	Borderline	Fail
Information gathering:		
Pass	Borderline	Fail
Applied clinical knowledge:		
Pass	Borderline	Fail

Notes for Marking

Patient safety

- Involves patient in the process (e.g. encouraging them to express their ideas, or preferences
- Negotiates a mutually agreed acceptable, safe, plan
- Does not enter into an agreement that could place the patient or operating surgeons in a difficult situation when she is under anaesthetic
- Demonstrates practice that is compliant with the Montgomery ruling

Communication with patient

- Greets patient and obtains patient's name and Introduces self, role
- Assesses starting point: ideas, concerns, and expectations
- Explains the procedure planned, using attentive listening—does this procedure match what she is expecting? Gives clear signposting
- Chunks and checks, using patient's response to guide next steps
- Gives explanation in an organized manner (signposting/summarising)
- Uses clear language, avoids jargon and confusing language
- Recognizes, acknowledges and validates patient's concerns and feelings (e.g. uses empathy)
- Appropriate non-verbal behaviour e.g. eye contact, posture, and position, movement, facial expression, use of voice (pace, tone)
- Calming and reassuring in approach to a difficult patient
- Provides support: e.g. concern, understanding, willingness to help
- Points towards information sources such as the Endometriosis UK support group

Information gathering

- Obtains a short, focused and relevant gynaecological history
- Assesses the patient's main concerns

Applied clinical knowledge

- Demonstrates a sound and comprehensive evidence-based clinical knowledge of the appropriate management of endometriosis that has yet to be confirmed laparoscopically
- Explains that the main aim of the surgery is to confirm the diagnosis and establish the extent of the disease
- Treatment with ovarian cystectomy could be appropriate though has a higher risk of recurrence than oophorectomy
- The extent of endometriosis could be so severe that it prevents any surgery on the day of operation and may be used to plan future operations, perhaps in combination with other specialties
- The operation may be able to treat the immediate problem (such as cystectomy/oophorectomy) but may require longer term management with drug therapy or further surgery
- The procedure—port sites, length of stay and recovery period are discussed appropriately
- The risks of laparoscopic surgery are discussed in a structured fashion with common risks of surgery (pain, bleeding, infection, thrombosis) as well as risk of laparotomy and damage to other organs
- The risk of death should also be covered
- The implications of not performing the operation should also be covered

Communication with patient

- Greets patient and obtains patient's name and introduces self, role
- Ability to take a short, relevant history
- Assesses starting point: ideas, concerns, and expectations
- Explains the procedure planned, using attentive listening—does this procedure match what she is expecting? Gives clear signposting
- Chunks and checks, using patient's response to guide next steps
- Gives explanation in an organized manner (signposting/summarising)
- Uses clear language, avoids jargon and confusing language
- Recognizes, acknowledges and validates patient's concerns and feelings (e.g. uses empathy)
- Appropriate non-verbal behaviour e.g. eye contact, posture and position, movement, facial expression, use of voice (pace, tone)
- Calming and reassuring in approach to a difficult patient
- Provides support: e.g. concern, understanding, willingness to help
- Points towards information sources such as Endometriosis UK support group

Further reading

Obtaining valid Consent, RCOG Clinical Governance Advice No. 6 January 2015, https://www.rcog.org.uk/globalassets/documents/guidelines/clinical-governance-advice/cga6.pdf

Chapter 6 **Core surgical skills**

Task 1 **Decision making**

Instructions for Candidate

This task assesses the following clinical skills:

- Patient safety
- Communication with patients and their relatives
- Information gathering
- Applied clinical knowledge

Sarah Bener is a 28-year-old lady in her second pregnancy.

She has had an elective caesarean section in her last pregnancy for a breech delivery two years ago.

She has no other health problems and her pregnancy has progressed well so far.

She is currently 36 weeks pregnant and has presented to the antenatal clinic to discuss the mode of delivery.

You have 10 minutes for this task (+ 2mins initial reading time)

Instruction for Assessors

Please read instructions to candidate and actor.

This station assesses the candidate's ability to come to a shared decision after discussing the pros and cons of both the options.

Please do not interrupt or prompt.

Record your overall clinical impression of the candidate for each domain (e.g. should this performance be pass, borderline or a fail).

Instructions for Role Player

You are Sarah Bener, a 28-year-old house wife.

You are 36 weeks pregnant. You are healthy and so far your pregnancy had progressed smoothly.

You feel good baby movements. The screening test as well as the baby's scan at 20 weeks has been normal.

You have one child, Imogen, born by caesarean section two years ago. It was an elective caesarean section as Imogen was in breech position. They did try turning her (ECV), but was unsuccessful. You were very much looking forward to a normal delivery and were disappointed that you needed a caesarean section.

The caesarean section was straightforward, without any complications. But you needed a few days to recover at home.

You are keen to have a normal delivery this time, but want to know the options and risks of the mode of delivery. Both you and your husband have always wanted a large family, so want to know the implications of a second section.

If the candidate does not mention VBAC, say that you have heard of this and can they explain more about it.

Temperament: You think you are mostly a calm, level-headed woman, but you do like to be organized and in control of things.

Ideas: You are hoping that you have a normal delivery this time around.

Concerns: You want what is best for the baby, but are keen to avoid a caesarean section. Your husband's work requires him to travel a lot away from home, so you are also required to look after Imogen. You are concerned that if you need a caesarean section, then it will be difficult for you to look after Imogen and the new baby. Your husband may be able to take a few days off, but you do not have any other family support.

Expectations: You want the student to explain:

- What are your options for delivery? Are they safe?
- What is VBAC? What are the advantages and disadvantages of attempting a vaginal Birth? How likely is it to be successful?
- Where will you need to deliver? Can you deliver at home?
- What are the advantages and disadvantages of undergoing another caesarean section? If you have a caesarean section this time, will it have implications on your next pregnancy?

Assessment

Marking Scheme

Patient safety:

Pass Borderline Fail

Communication with patients and their relatives:

Pass Borderline Fail

Information gathering:

Pass Borderline Fail

Applied clinical knowledge:

Pass Borderline Fail

Notes for Marking

Patient safety

- Confirms no contraindication to VBAC
- Assesses the patient's main concerns and ideas
- Gives options and discusses the pros and cons of VBAC and LSCS
- Discusses possible complications and monitoring
- Involves patient in the process (e.g. encouraging them to express their ideas, or preferences
- Negotiates a mutually agreed acceptable, safe, plan

Communication with patients and their relatives

- Greets, introduces self and role, checks patient's name
- Consent to proceed and explains nature of interview

- Assesses patient's starting point (what the patient wants to know) and sets the agenda
- Clear organized explanation in logical sequence
- Chunks: e.g. provides information in reasonable chunks
- Checks patient understands.
- Language (easily understood, avoids or explains jargon)
- Uses visual aids appropriately e.g. diagrams or uses analogies to aid explanation
- Presents a clear and succinct history to the assessor

Information gathering

- Obtains a relevant obstetric history
- Obtains views on mode of delivery

Applied clinical knowledge

Demonstrates a sound and comprehensive evidence-based clinical knowledge—e.g. provides evidence-based facts about VBAC. Discusses both options of VBAC and elective caesarean section with pros and cons.

In counselling Sarah, the candidates must include the following:

Confirms had a straightforward intra-operative and postoperative period during the last LSCS
Explain options of having a vaginal birth or a caesarean delivery
Either choice is safe with different risks and benefits. Overall, both are safe choices with only very small risks

Option 1—VBAC

Is attempting vaginal delivery after a caesarean section
Overall, about three out of four women (75%) with a straightforward pregnancy who go into labour give birth vaginally following one caesarean delivery
The advantages of a successful VBAC include a vaginal birth a shorter recovery and a shorter stay in hospital less abdominal pain after birth of having surgery a greater chance of an uncomplicated normal birth in future pregnancies. The disadvantages of VBAC include scar weakening or scar rupture, emergency caesarean delivery, risks to the baby, blood transfusion and infection in the uterus
Sarah will be advized to deliver in hospital so that an emergency caesarean delivery can be carried out if necessary
During labour, the baby and the progress of the labour will be closely monitored

Option 2—Elective LSCS

The advantages of elective repeat caesarean delivery include virtually no risk of uterine scar rupture; it avoids the risks of labour and particularly the risk of possible brain damage or stillbirth from lack of oxygen during labour, knowledge of the date of delivery
The disadvantages of elective repeat caesarean delivery include, a longer and possibly more difficult operation. Chance of a blood clot (thrombosis). There is a longer recovery period. Breathing problems for your baby, risks of surgery like bleeding, infection, trauma to surrounding structures, a need for elective caesarean delivery in future pregnancies, possibility of the placenta growing into the scar making it difficult to remove at caesarean (placenta accreta or percreta).
Comes to a shared agreement

Notes for Candidate

The scenario is taken from a common clinical scenario of our daily practice. It not only assesses the process of communication but also assesses the content of the knowledge given to the patient. It is important *how* you provide the information to the patient.

Practice this scenario with one of your friends who can act as a role player and ask another friend to provide you with feedback.

Further reading

Green top Guideline Birth after caesarean birth https://www.rcog.org.uk/globalassets/documents/guidelines/gtg_45.pdf

Task 2 **Laparoscopic entry technique**

Instructions for candidate

This task assesses the following clinical skills:

- Patient safety
- Communication with patients and their relatives
- Information gathering
- Applied clinical knowledge

Ruth Mason is a 38-year-old lady with a BMI of 40.

She has been complaining of lower abdomen dull ache and an ultrasound scan has indicated a 6cms dermoid cyst on her left ovary. She is booked for laparoscopic left salpingoopherectomy.

In the past she had a midline laparotomy and bowel resection secondary to Crohn's disease under the surgeons. You are seeing her in the preoperative clinic to obtain consent for the procedure to explain the procedure and the risks. You do not have to obtain a written consent.

You have 10 minutes for this task (+ 2mins initial reading time).

Instruction for Assessors

Please read instructions to candidate and actor.

This task assesses the candidate's ability to apply knowledge in relation to laparoscopy in a lady with previous abdominal surgeries. It also assesses their communication skills to be able to give relevant information and obtain consent.

Please do not prompt or interrupt the candidate.

Record your overall clinical impression of the candidate for each domain (e.g. should this performance be pass, borderline or a fail).

Instructions for Role Player

You are Ruth Mason, a 38-year-old school teacher.

You were diagnosed with Crohn's disease in your teens. This required bowel resection with re-anastomosis two years back. Your bowel symptoms are well controlled presently.

You had two children in the past both normal vaginal deliveries. Presently you are using barrier method for contraception.

You have been having dull lower abdominal ache and your GP organized an ultrasound scan which indicated a 6cm dermoid cyst on the left ovary.

You saw the gynaecology consultant who has listed you for laparoscopic removal of the left ovary and tube.

You are worried about having another operation because of the past history and bowel problems but at the same time wanted to have the cyst removed as you have been told that the cyst can twist or burst in the abdomen.

You have come for pre-operative assessment and the doctor will be taking your consent for the scheduled operation.

Temperament: You are very apprehensive and scared.

Ideas: You are hoping that everything will go well and you will go home the same day.

Concerns: You want to know how you will enter the abdomen. You don't like the big scar on your tummy and keen to avoid another big cut. Your husband may be able to take a few days off, but you do not have any other family support if you need prolonged hospitalization.

Expectations: You want the doctor to explain:

- How will you gain access into the tummy?
- Will this damage her internal organs? What percentage of cases has damage to the bowel?
- What are the other complications?

Assessment

Marking Scheme		
Patient safety:		
Pass	Borderline	Fail
Communication with patients and their relatives:		
Pass	Borderline	Fail
Information gathering:		
Pass	Borderline	Fail
Applied clinical knowledge:		
Pass	Borderline	Fail

Notes for Marking

Patient safety

- Assesses the patient's main concerns and ideas
- Gives options and discusses the pros and cons different entry techniques
- Discusses possible complications and how to reduce the risk of complications
- Involves patient in the process (e.g. encouraging them to express their ideas, or preferences
- Negotiates a mutually agreed acceptable, safe, plan

Communication with patients and their relatives

- Greets, introduces self and role, checks patient's name
- Consent to proceed and explains nature of interview
- Assesses patient's starting point (what the patient wants to know) and sets the agenda
- Clear organized explanation in logical sequence
- Chunks: e.g. provides information in reasonable chunks
- Checks patient's understanding
- Language (easily understood, avoids or explains jargon)
- Uses visual aids appropriately e.g. diagrams or uses analogies to aid explanation
- Presents a clear and succinct history to the assessor

Information gathering

- Obtains a focussed and relevant gynaecological history
- Obtains a relevant previous surgical history

Applied clinical knowledge

Demonstrates a sound and comprehensive evidence-based clinical knowledge—e.g. in counselling Ms Mason, the candidates must include the following:

1. Almost one-third of patients with previous surgery through a midline incision will be at risk of injury from the primary trocar if it is inserted at the umbilical site. In over half of these patients, the adhesions involved the bowel.
2. In such a situation, a closed Veress needle technique or visual entry technique at palmer's point may have advantages over open entry.
3. In cases such as these open laparoscopy does succeed in virtually eliminating type I injuries to the bowel and major vessels it does not eliminate the risk of type II bowel damage. Possibly, this is because the method does not allow recognition of bowel adhesions prior to direct cut down.
4. Complications arising from laparoscopy are often related to initial entry into the abdomen. Life-threatening complications include injury to viscera e.g. the bowel or bladder, or to vasculature e.g. major abdominal and anterior abdominal wall vessels.
5. General risks of anaesthesia and surgery:
   - Venous thromboembolism
   - Atelectasis leading to infection
   - MI or CVA
   - Death
6. Procedure specific risks:
   - Haemorrhage resulting in transfusion, re-operation, prolonged stay in hospital
   - Damage to other organs, resulting in further surgery and a longer recovery time
   - Infection secondary to collections requiring reoperation and or drainage with prolonged hospitalization
   - Adhesions formation resulting in bowel complications, further surgery and prolonged hospitalization
   - The insufflation gas may give pain and other complications
   - Keloid scar formation
   - Hernia formation at the wound site
   - In obese patients and smokers, more wound and chest infection, heart and lung complications and venous thromboembolism
   - Fistula formation

Notes for Candidate

The scenario is taken from a common clinical scenario of our daily practice. It not only assesses the process of communication but also assesses the content of the knowledge given to the patient. It is important *how* you provide the information to the patient.

Practice this scenario with one of your friends who can act as a role player and ask another friend to provide you with feedback.

Further reading

Ahmad G, Duffy JMN, Phillips K, Watson A. Laparoscopic entry techniques. *Cochrane Database of Systematic Reviews,* 2008; (1): CD006583.

Jansen FW, Kolkman W, Bakkum EA, de Kroon CD, Trimbos-Kemper TC, Trimbos JB. Complications of laparoscopy: an inquiry about closed- versus open-entry technique. *American Journal of Obstetrics & Gynecology* 2004; 190: 634–8.

Chapter 7 **Post-operative care**

Task 1 **Recognising and dealing with postoperative complication**

Instructions for Candidate

This task assesses the following clinical skills:

- Patient safety
- Communication with colleagues
- Applied clinical knowledge

You are the ST5 on duty. Your ST1 who is taking her first on-call in the department has just received a phone call from the out-of-hours surgery, and you have accepted to see this lady in the emergency. She had a laparoscopy done three days ago, for suspected endometriosis. Now, she presented with right sided loin pain and mild fever. The GP thinks she is significantly tender in her right loin on examination. You have advised to bring her in to rule out ureteric injury. Your ST1 wants to discuss this case with you before the patient arrives in emergency.

You are expected to answer the questions of the trainee and demonstrate your teaching skills.

You have 10 minutes for this task (+ 2mins initial reading time).

Instructions for Assessor

Please read the instructions to candidate and the actor. Allow the candidate to conduct the interview undisturbed unless they are straying off the track of the question (in which case you can show them their instructions again).

This conversation is going to be among two professionals where the ST5 should demonstrate the following teaching skills:

- Ability to set objectives and structure the session.
- Establish the background knowledge of the learner
- Identify their learning needs
- Use appropriate diagrams or refer to appropriate reference readings/evidence to support teaching
- Allow the ST1 to make contribution in the discussion, invite questions, check understanding, address concerns and facilitate learning by giving some relevant task
- Give feedback and gather feedback
- Plan a follow-up meeting to check learning

Record your overall clinical impression of the candidate for each domain (e.g. should this performance be pass, borderline, or a fail).

Instructions for Role Player

You are the SHO and want to discuss this case with your registrar before she arrives in the emergency. You have joined the department a week ago, and this is your first on-call shift. You were present in the theatre at the time of this procedure and know that it was a complicated procedure because of presence of adhesions. But her post-operative recovery was uneventful and she was discharged home on the next day. You are a bit unsure how she can sustain a ureteric injury because you think nothing was done to the ureters. Ask your registrar the following questions?

- How will you confirm the diagnosis?
- What will be her management if she has a ureteric injury? Will she require a re-operation?
- How will you explain this to the patient?
- Was this avoidable?
- Anything that can be done to minimize risk of such complications?

Temperament: You are a very enthusiastic SHO and want to be well aware of what you will be doing with regards to management. You also want to know how to explain the situation to the patient.

Ideas: You are expecting it to be a bit challenging to deal with this patient, as she was not an easy person to deal with during her previous admission.

Concerns: You have concerns that the patient may raise a complaint and you want to know if this injury was avoidable, what can be done in future for such cases to avoid these kind of injuries etc.

Expectations: You want to fill up gaps in your knowledge and be confident while dealing with this patient in the emergency room.

Assessment

Marking Scheme

Patient safety:
Pass Borderline Fail

Communication with colleague:
Pass Borderline Fail

Information gathering:
Pass Borderline Fail

Applied clinical knowledge:
Pass Borderline Fail

Notes for Marking

Patient safety

- Discusses consent process and patient information leaflets on frequent and serious risks of the procedure
- Emphasizes the importance of meticulous documentation on each occasion i.e. clinic notes, pre-operative assessment, consent, operative notes and follow-up plans
- Explains the importance of completing an incident form

- Discussing the case in departmental meeting and identifying areas of improvement in safer practice
- Explains the complaint process if patient is unhappy with the explanation and care

Communication with the colleague

- Greets, appropriate introduction mentioning level of training and establishes level of training of the learner
- Creates rapport with less experienced colleague
- Explains agenda of the meeting and checks her agenda
- Determine her learning needs (what she wants to learn) and expectations from the teaching session (is she finding anything particularly challenging to deal with)
- Establish her existing knowledge
- Clear organized explanation in logical sequence Chunks: e.g. provides information in reasonable chunks colleague's understanding. Language (checks if she is unfamiliar with any term)
- Uses visual aids appropriately e.g. diagrams or uses analogies to aid explanation, provide reading references
- Give and gather feedback
- Arrange a follow-up meeting
- Encourages the trainee to be open and honest about procedure and possible complications
- Provides with information about the person performing the procedure and safeguard in place e.g. competent clinician or junior doctor under direct supervision
- Explain mechanism in place to deal with complications and learn from such complication
- Being honest about further investigations, repeat hospital admission, need of MDT and a further intervention depending on the nature of injury

Applied clinical knowledge

- Demonstrates a sound and comprehensive evidence-based clinical knowledge—e.g. explains delayed presentation is likely to be due to transmission of electric energy to the adjacent tissues. Electrodamage can cause necrosis which can result in extravasation of urine; electrodamage to ureteric adventitia can cause ischemic strictures leading to ureteric obstruction and hydronephrosis.
- More than 70% of the time, unilateral ureteral injury is noticed postoperatively, when the patient may present with flank pain, prolonged ileus, fever, watery vaginal discharge, or elevated serum creatinine levels. In cases of bilateral ureteral injury, anuria is the first clinical sign.

Notes for Candidate

The scenario is taken from a common clinical scenario of our daily practice. It not only assesses the process of communication but also assesses the content of the knowledge required for teaching a junior colleague. It is important how you provide the information to your junior colleague who has just joined the speciality.

Practice this scenario with one of your friends who can act as a role player and ask another friend to provide you with feedback.

Further reading

Gopinath, D. and Jha, S., Urological complications following gynaecological surgery, Obstetrics, *Gynaecology & Reproductive Medicine*, 23; (11): 337–42.

Hogg, S. and Milliken D., Avoiding and managing complications in gynaecological surgery, *Obstetrics, Gynaecology & Reproductive Medicine*, 23; (3): 81–7.

Task 2 **Postoperative management**

Instructions for Candidates

This task assesses the following clinical skills:

- Patient safety
- Communication with patients and their relatives
- Information gathering
- Applied clinical knowledge

You are the night Registrar on call. At around 6:30, you are asked to see Margaret Bultoph.

Miss Bultoph is a 49-year-old woman who has had a Laparoscopic Bilateral salpingo-oophorectomy for a right persistent ovarian cyst, around 40hrs ago (day three) in the day procedure unit.

This was a straightforward procedure completed in 30 minutes and the plan was to discharge the patient home once she was comfortable and had passed urine. She was to be discharged home on Paracetamol and combined cyclical HRT. She had been counselled regarding the latter.

However, Margaret's pain had not been controlled and she had required multiple pain relief medications. She was not comfortable enough to be discharged and had been admitted to the gynaecology unit after closure of the day procedure unit at 8.00pm on the day. The on call doctor that reviewed her and was satisfied that there was no ongoing bleeding or visceral injury.

She had also required an indwelling catheter.

She had remained haemodynamically stable but resistant to mobilization as she was worried about the pain coming back and still has the indwelling catheter, the plan was to remove the catheter at 6.00 am today. The nurse went to do the same, when Margaret complained of right sided chest pain and feeling breathless.

At 6.00 am her observations are:

- Pulse—102
- BP—110/64
- RR—22
- O_2 sats—93% on air
- Temp—37.6 C

On examination, you find her respiratory system, unremarkable, apart from the tachypnoea.

Her drug chart has the following medications:

- Dihydrocodeine 60mg QDS
- Diclofenac 75mg 12hrly
- PRN Oromorph
- Cyclical HRT

Your task is to:

- Organize the necessary investigations and initiate the management
- explain the investigations, results and diagnosis to the patient and answer her questions

You have 10 minutes for this task (+ 2mins initial reading time).

Instructions for Assessor

This task assesses the candidates' ability to organize relevant investigations and manage pulmonary embolism.

It also assesses their communication skills. Firstly to explain the investigations, results and management to the patient, but also the fact that she should have been started on prophylactic Dalteparin (Heparin) when she was admitted.

They should stop her HRT.

Please give them the following results (Table 7.1, Box 7.1–7.3) only after they have asked for the investigation. If they ask for V-Q scan, tell them it is not available in their place of work, as they should ask for CTPA in this patient.

Table 7.1 ABG results

Date xx/xx/xxxx
Margaret Bultoph
Date of Birth: dd/mm/yy
Hospital no: xyx
Sample taken on room air (21%):

		(Normal Range)
pO_2	**9.6 kPa**	11–15
pCO_2	**3.5 kPa**	4.5–6
pH	7.40	7.35–7.45

Box 7.1 CTPA results

Margaret Bultoph
Date of Birth: dd/mm/yy
Hospital no: xyx
Conclusion:
The CTPA shows evidence of a showing a 'saddle embolus' at the bifurcation of the pulmonary artery and thrombus burden in the lobar branches of both main pulmonary arteries.

Box 7.2 D-Dimer results

Margaret Bultoph
Date of Birth: dd/mm/yy
Hospital no: xyx
400ng/ml
Note- A D-Dimer of <230ng/ml, together with a low clinical suspicion (score) of VTE, significantly reduces the likelihood of DVT (in non-anticoagulated patients).

Box 7.3 Other results

Normal full blood count, renal and liver function tests
ECG—Normal.
X-ray Chest—Normal

Instructions for Role Player

You are Margaret Bultoph a 49-year-old. You work in a bank.

You live alone with your two cats and have recently moved to this town.

You were admitted three days ago in the day procedure unit for removal of your ovaries. You were known to have a right sided 6cms ovarian cyst for the last six months. This was noted on a scan performed six months ago when you had presented to your GP with right sided pelvic pain. The pain was never severe and subsided on its own. The specialist at the hospital had therefore suggested that a scan be repeated in three months. This scan had shown that the cyst was still the same. Your blood tests called tumour markers were normal and this was a simple cyst.

You had elected that you undergo surgery to remove this cyst. You were offered removal of both your ovaries given your age. Your mother had died of cancer of the ovary and so you agreed.

This was to be done as day case and you were going to ask your neighbour to look in on you.

You have lived alone since your mother died five years ago. You are independent and do not like to bother anyone.

You have not undergone any surgery before nor have any medical problems. You are not allergic to any medications.

At your pre assessment, you were asked if there was any one to look after you at home and you had said that your neighbour would, as you did not want to leave your cats in the cattery.

However, after the surgery, you were in pain and did not feel you could go home. The worst was the catheter. There was no way you were going to go home with the catheter.

You had been counselled re the HRT and were very keen to have the HRT as otherwise you felt; you could not cope with your work.

After admission and the pain medications, the pain subsided.

On the third day, you suddenly developed pain in your chest on the right and every time you took in a breath, it hurt you more. You were breathless. You have no cough or any other symptoms.

You expect the candidate to explain how each investigation is done, why and what will it show.

After the candidate organizes the necessary tests, they should explain what pulmonary embolism means.

When they have finished explaining to you, if they have not volunteered and performed the duty of candour, ask-whether you should have been given injections to thin the blood as your mother had after her surgery?

If they have spontaneously not done so, then ask why did you develop this?

How will you be managed? Short and long term?

Assessment

Marking Scheme

Patient safety:

Pass	Borderline	Fail

Communication with patients and their relatives:

Pass	Borderline	Fail

Information gathering:

Pass	Borderline	Fail

Applied clinical knowledge:

Pass	Borderline	Fail

Notes for Marking

Patient safety

- Stops HRT
- Involves patient in the process (e.g. encouraging them to express their ideas, or preferences
- Keeps patient informed throughout the process
- Performs duty of candour
- Is open, honest and non-defensive
- Apologizes for complication
- Explains that there will be an investigation into whether the complication could have been prevented
- Explains that patient will be told outcome of this investigation
- Explains that will be given contact details for someone to contact regarding the investigation
- Explains her thromboprophylaxis should have been reviewed when she was admitted and again the next day

Communication with patients and their relatives

- Introduces themselves
- Explains why they are reviewing the patient
- Explains the investigations using lay terminology
- Explains the results and further investigations
- Explains the management
- Clear organized explanation in logical sequence
- Chunks: i.e. provides information in reasonable chunks
- Checks patient's understanding.
- Language (easily understood, avoids or explains jargon)
- Uses visual aids appropriately e.g. diagrams or uses analogies to aid explanation

Information gathering

- Obtains a short and focussed pre operative history
- Obtains a short and focussed post operative history

Applied clinical knowledge

- Correctly identifies the high possibility of pulmonary embolism
- Arranges the relevant investigations-ABG, ECG,X-Ray Chest, CTPA
- Interprets the ABG correctly
- Initiates the correct management
- Oxygen
- Therapeutic doses of heparin/dalteparin/tinzaperin/enoxaperin
- STOPS the HRT

Further reading

Nice Guidelines, Pulmonary embolism, January 2015, http://cks.nice.org.uk/pulmonary-embolism

Chapter 8 **Surgical procedures**

Task 1 **Electrocautery and electro-diathermy**

Instructions for Candidate

This task assesses the following clinical skills:

- Patient safety
- Communication with colleagues
- Applied clinical knowledge

Mrs. Ahmed is a 48-year-old lady undergoing total abdominal hysterectomy and bilateral salpingo-oophorectomy for heavy menstrual bleeding with a 20 week size fibroid. She is generally well and has undergone a left hip replacement five years ago.

Your consultant has asked you to commence the surgery by opening the abdomen with a vertical subumbilical incision. She will shortly join you for the surgery. The Foundation Year 1 doctor will be assisting you in the interim.

You will be presented with scenarios in the theatre. Your task is to problem solve and answer the queries of the F1 doctor.

You have 10 minutes for this task (+ 2mins initial reading time).

Instructions for Assessor

There is no role player for this scenario.

This scenario checks the understanding of Monopolar diathermy and the ability to problem solve. It also assesses the understanding of safety issues surrounding electrocautery.

First tell the candidate:

The Theatre Assistant Practitioner (ODP) is newly qualified and normally works in the ENT theatres. You start the incision using a finger switch diathermy but it is not working

What will you do?

The candidate should first check if the machine is on

Tell them that is was not on, but has now been switched on

As soon as the machine is switched on, the machine starts beeping

What should the ODP do next?

If the candidate asks if there are any indications on the machine, say the sign of the returning electrodes is highlighted

The candidate should check if the returning electrodes (pads) have been applied.

They had not been. The ODP asks where he should apply the returning electrodes.

The candidates should ask the electrode to be placed on the right buttock.

The ODP asks if it is OK to put the returning electrode on the left buttock as the scrub nurse and trolley are on the right and it is convenient to apply on the left.

The candidate should explain that as Mrs. Ahmed has had a hip replacement on the left, it is important to avoid applying the returning electrode near the metal implant and the scarring around it, for safety.

The ODP asks that he has never seen a split returning electrode. Why is it split?

The candidate should say that the split electrode is introduced to minimize the risk of burns at the site of application of the returning electrode. If the electrode is not applied properly, decreasing the area of the returning energy, this concentrates the current over a small area and can cause severe burns. With the split electrode, an interrogation current constantly checks the quality of contact between the patient and the patient returning electrode. If there is a breach in the contact between the patient and the patient returning electrode, then the generator automatically stops.

The ODP applies the PRE (Patient Returning Electrode) on the Right buttock of the patient. The diathermy still does not work. The ODP asks if he should increase the power/voltage?

The candidate should say no to increase in the power/voltag**e.**

They should ask the ODP to check if the PRE is applied correctly.

The ODP checks and as it was not applied correctly, affixes the PRE correctly this time. The finger switch now starts working.

The F1 doctor assists you in the abdominal incision and your consultant takes you through the hysterectomy.

After the surgery, the F1 doctor has some questions for you.

Could you explain to him, how through the same current, you could use the diathermy for cutting ad coagulating. He heard you say, you wanted a blend and on spray. What does it mean? When do you use these options?

There are two options in monopolar diathermy: Cut (Yellow) and 'Coag'/Coagulation (Blue).

Cut (Yellow button) the cutting action of monopolar diathermy is achieved by a continuous electric current waveform action which vaporizes the tissues on contact. This allows cutting of tissues without coagulation. The 'Cut' setting has two settings called 'Pure' and 'Blend' depending on the levels of energy involved.

Coagulation or 'Coag' (Blue button) This uses the same alternating current but the waveform is only on 6% of the time. This allows coagulation of tissues while cutting. 'Coag' can be used directly through the active electrode or through a conducting device such as insulated forceps to direct the coagulation more accurately. As with 'Cut' there are two modes: desiccation (also called 'forced coag') and fulguration.

Desiccation ('Forced Coag') this allows more precise coagulation and the electrode needs to be in touch with the target tissue. The voltages are somewhat lower in desiccation mode compared to Fulguration but with slightly higher currents (0.5W vs 0.1W).

Fulguration ('Spray Coag') this is good for haemostasis and 'sprays' a shower of sparks a few millimetre away from the targeted tissue. It is achieved by using very high voltages (around 6000V) with lower currents. It should be avoided on delicate organs like bowel and near large vessels as the effect is less controlled than desiccation and can cause thermal injuries. This is typically used in subcutaneous tissue.

Record your overall clinical impression of the candidate for each domains (i.e. should this performance be pass, borderline, or a fail).

Assessment

Marking Scheme

Patient safety:

Pass Borderline Fail

Communication with colleagues:

Pass Borderline Fail

Applied clinical knowledge:

Pass Borderline Fail

Notes for Marking

Patient safety

- Aware of the importance of the split pad
- Aware not to increase the power/voltage of the diathermy if not working and making the other safety checks
- Aware when not to use the spray
- Honest
- Says will seek senior input when does not know the answer

Communication with colleagues

- Confident
- Clearly able to give instructions to the ODP
- When explaining the F1 doctor, explains in a logical manner

Applied clinical knowledge

- Has a robust knowledge of electrodiathermy

Further reading

Electrosurgery, Stratog, https://stratog.rcog.org.uk/tutorial/general-principles/electrosurgery-6040
Basic Practical Skills in Obstetrics and gynaecology, *Participant manual*, RCOG, Cambridge University press.

Task 2 **Hysterectomy**

Instructions for Candidate

This task assesses the following clinical skills:

- Patient safety
- Communication with patients and their relatives
- Information gathering
- Applied clinical knowledge

You are an ST5 doctor working in a gynaecology clinic with your consultant. Your consultant has asked you to see a follow up patient, Patricia Simmonds who is a 45-year-old dental receptionist.

She is coming back to see you having tried various medical options for her menorrhagia, none of which have helped and she wishes to discuss the next options available to her.

You will be given the examination findings and asked some questions by the assessor.

Your task is to:

- Take a brief history
- Explain the options available to her
- Explain the associated risks and complications
- Answer any of her questions

You have 10 minutes for this task (+ 2mins initial reading time).

Instructions for Assessor

Please read instruction to candidate and role player.

Allow the candidate to conduct the interview undisturbed unless they are straying off the track of the question (in which case you can show them their instructions again).

Once the candidate has taken a relevant history and presented to you, provide the candidate with following information.

Abdominal examination—unremarkable
Speculum examination—cervix satisfactory
Bimanual examination—normal sized, mobile, anteverted uterus, no adnexal masses or tenderness, mild apical descent

Now ask the candidate to explain the management plan to Mrs Simmonds. The candidate should discuss hysterectomy and the potential routes, the patient would be a candidate for vaginal hysterectomy.

There are some marks on the process mark sheet for the actor to assign at the end of the station.

Record your overall clinical impression of the candidate for each domains (i.e. should this performance be pass, borderline, or a fail).

Instruction for Role Player

You are Patricia Simmonds, a 45-year-old dental receptionist. For the last few years your periods have become increasingly heavy and they are now impacting significantly on your life and you are looking for a definitive solution now.

You have had two children, both born vaginally, now aged 17 and 15.

You are otherwise fit and well and have had no previous operations.

You have tried medical treatment including a coil, but none of these options have helped you and you are now at the end of your tether as you bleed very heavy for five days a month, and then feel exhausted.

You want to know what the options are, what the associated risks are and what your recovery will be like.

Temperament: You think you are a calm, level headed woman who can take in information rationally.

Ideas: You have read some information on the internet and you remember your mother had a hysterectomy, you don't remember much more, but you know she was out of action for a while after.

Concerns: you are concerned that this will get worse if surgery isn't offered.

Expectations: You want to be offered surgical management.

You want the doctor to explain the following:

Risks of surgery, recovery time, success rates, and length of stay in hospital.

Assessment

Marking Scheme

Patient safety:

Pass Borderline Fail

Communication with patients and their relatives:

Pass Borderline Fail

Information gathering:

Pass Borderline Fail

Applied clinical knowledge:

Pass Borderline Fail

Notes for Marking

Patient safety

- Assesses the patient's main concerns and ideas
- Gives options and discusses the pros and cons of different management plans
- Discusses possible complications and measures to reduce them
- Involves patient in the process (e.g. encouraging them to express their ideas, or preferences
- Negotiates a mutually agreed acceptable, safe, plan
- Open and honest about procedure and possible complications
- Provides patient with information about the person performing the procedure and safeguard in place i.e. competent clinician or junior doctor under direct supervision. Explains mechanism in place to deal with complications and learn from complications
- Is honest about prolongation of recovery time if untoward complication happen

Communication with patients and their relatives

- Greets, introduces self and role, checks patient's name
- Consent to proceed and explains nature of interview
- Assesses patient's starting point (what the patient wants to know) and sets the agenda

- Clear organized explanation in logical sequence
- Chunks: i.e. provides information in reasonable chunks
- Checks patient's understanding.
- Language (easily understood, avoids or explains jargon)
- Uses visual aids appropriately e.g. diagrams or uses analogies to aid explanation
- Presents a clear and succinct history to the assessor

Information gathering

- Obtains a relevant and focused history

Applied clinical knowledge

- This patient has menorrhagia and the history should include:
  - the extent, duration and inconvenience caused by the symptoms
  - treatment options tried thus far
  - obstetric history—number of children, mode of delivery, birth weights
  - smear history
  - family planning issues
  - PMH and PSH
  - family history, social history, and current drug history
- Demonstrates a sound and comprehensive evidence-based clinical knowledge
- Offers hysterectomy
- Discusses various routes of hysterectomy
- Discusses advantages and disadvantages of each route
- Recommends the least invasive route with quicker recovery

Further reading

AAGL Advancing Minimally Invasive Gynecology Worldwide, AAGL Position Statement: Route of Hysterectomy to Treat Benign Uterine Disease, *Journal of Minimally Invasive Gynecology*, 2011. 18; (1). http://www.aagl.org/wp-content/uploads/2013/03/aagl-hysterectomy-position-statement.pdf

ACOG Committee Opinion No. 444, Choosing the Route of Hysterectomy for Benign Disease, 2009. http://www.acog.org/-/media/Committee-Opinions/Committee-on-Gynecologic-Practice/co444.pdf?dmc=1

DeLancey JOL, Skinner BD, Selecting the route for hysterectomy: A structured approach, *Contemporary OB/GYN*, 2013. http://contemporaryobgyn.modernmedicine.com/contemporary-obgyn/content/tags/gynecologic-surgery/selecting-route-hysterectomy-structured-approach?page=full

Chapter 9 **Antenatal Care**

Task 1 **Pre-conception counselling**

Instructions for Candidate

This task assesses the following clinical skills:

- Patient safety
- Communication with patients and their relatives
- Information gathering
- Applied clinical knowledge

Mrs Yvonne Williams is 29-year-old nulliparous woman with Type 1 diabetes and BMI of 39 and has been referred by her GP to the hospital clinic for pre-pregnancy counselling and advice. Her diabetes is poorly controlled and she is planning a pregnancy in the near future. Following discussions with her community midwife. Mrs Williams is aware that with her health condition, pregnancy and delivery carries a higher risk but she would welcome an opportunity to discuss her concerns with an obstetrician.

Mrs Williams will be asking you certain questions which you should try to answer and explain, for example:

- What are the risks?
- What measures can be taken to reduce risk?
- What measures will be taken during pregnancy?

You have 10 minutes for this task (+ 2mins initial reading time).

Instructions for Assessor

This task assesses the candidate's ability to conduct a pre-pregnancy counselling. It tests their communication skills and application of knowledge regarding diabetes in pregnancy

Record your overall clinical impression of the candidate for each domain (e.g. should this performance be pass, borderline, or a fail).

Instructions for Role Player

You are Mrs Yvonne Williams is 29-year-old and have never been pregnant before. You have diabetes since childhood and you also struggle with your weight. You were last time told that your BMI is 39. You have been referred by her GP to the hospital clinic for pre-pregnancy counselling and advice. Your diabetes is poorly controlled and you are planning a pregnancy in the near future. Following discussion with your community midwife, you are aware that with her health condition pregnancy and delivery carries a higher risk but you welcome an opportunity to discuss your concerns with an obstetrician. You should ask the following questions to the candidate.

- What are the risks?
- What measures can be taken to reduce risk?
- What measures will be taken during pregnancy?

Temperament: You are careless about your health and have not thought about it seriously until your midwife brought up the discussion. You try to take your insulin

Ideas: You now have some idea that your weight and diabetes can have some serious implications on your and the baby's health.

Concerns: You have concerns that you may not be able to lose weight due to your diabetes and may not be able to achieve a good control of your blood sugar levels either.

Expectations: You are expecting to have a clear understanding of your health condition and its implications on the pregnancy, so that you can make a decision on the right time to conceive.

Assessment

Marking Scheme

Patient safety:

Pass	Borderline	Fail

Communication with patients and their relatives:

Pass	Borderline	Fail

Information gathering:

Pass	Borderline	Fail

Applied clinical knowledge:

Pass	Borderline	Fail

Notes for Marking

Patient safety

- Assesses the patient's main concerns and ideas on every stage and addresses them appropriately as previously mentioned. Revise medications, provides information on early booking and early investigations, emphasizes on the importance of compliance with follow-up and treatment
- Open and honest discussion about the implications of both conditions on her health, pregnancy and the new born. Provides with information on early booking and contact numbers

Communication with patients and their relatives

- Greets, appropriate introduction.
- Creates rapport with the patient
- Explains agenda of the meeting and checks her agenda
- Determine her existing understandings and explores her concerns
- Establish the causes of her being no-compliant to her treatment
- Clear organized explanation in logical sequence chunks: language avoids medical jargon
- Provides information leaflets
- Appropriate use of multidisciplinary team, diabetic clinics and other systems in place
- Demonstrates reliable counselling skills

Information gathering

- Obtains a relevant obstetric history
- Obtains a relevant history pertaining to diabetes
- Obtains views, expectations, and plans regarding pregnancy

Applied clinical knowledge

Demonstrates a sound and comprehensive evidence-based clinical knowledge—e.g. explains the implications in simple and clear language and emphasisis on the control of both conditions, i.e. weight and diabetes.

The following information should be covered under each question the role-player will ask.

What are the risks?

1. Maternal: thromboembolism, pre-eclampsia, anaesthetic complications, preterm labour, dysfunctional labour, increased chances of caesarean section, wound infection, postpartum haemorrhage
2. Fetal: miscarriage, congenital anomaly (including increased risk of neural tube defect), macrosomia, birth injury, perinatal mortality (including stillbirth and neonatal mortality)

What measures can be taken to reduce risk:

1. Gradual reduction in body weight to a BMI of <30 through dietetic measures (advice by a dietician), and lifestyle changes.
2. Control of blood glucose: Fasting (on waking up) 5 to 7mmol/L; 4 to 7micromol/L before meals at other times
3. HbA1c < 48mmol/mol. Monthly testing
4. Retinal assessment: retinopathy worsens in pregnancy. Assessment at regular intervals in pregnancy, usually at 16–20 weeks of gestation and again at 28 weeks
5. Renal assessment: Refer to nephrologist before stopping contraceptive if serum creatinine 120micromol/L or more. Urinary albumin/creatinine ratio >30mg/mmol. Glomerular filtration rate <45ml/min/1.73 m^2.
6. Medications:

   5mg daily folic acid starting one month before pregnancy until 12 weeks of gestation;

What measures will be taken during pregnancy?

1. Care and birth in a consultant led unit.
2. Medications:

   75mg aspirin from 12 weeks of gestation until birth of baby;

   10microgram vitamin D daily during pregnancy and breastfeeding.
3. Glucose control: fasting 5.3mmol or less; one hour after meal, not more than 7.8mmol; two hours after meal, not more than 6.4mmol.
4. Anaesthetic review. Only indicated if BMI 40 or more, but added risk is Type 1 diabetes poorly controlled.
5. Growth scans if clinical assessment unsatisfactory.
6. Active management of third stage.
7. Issues about manual handling and thromboprophylaxis if BMI 40 or more.

Notes for Candidate

The scenario is taken from a common clinical scenario of our daily practice. It not only assesses the process of communication but also assesses the content of the knowledge given to the patient. It is important how you provide the information to the patient.

Practice this scenario with one of your friends who can act as a role player and ask another friend to provide you with feedback.

Further reading

NICE guidance on the management of diabetes, https://www.nice.org.uk/guidance/ng3

Task 2 **Female Genital Mutilation**

Instructions for Candidate

This task assesses the following clinical skills:

- Patient safety
- Communication with patients and their relatives
- Information gathering
- Applied clinical knowledge

You are an ST-5 doctor working in an antenatal clinic with your consultant. Your next patient is Mrs Arayomi Adebola, 30 years old, who has been referred at 16 weeks gestation by her midwife for a positive history of female genital mutilation (FGM).

Your task is to:

- Take a relevant history
- Outline the legal and regulatory responsibilities to the patient
- Outline the antenatal management to the patient

You do not need to examine her. On completion of these tasks you will be given the examination findings. Please then formulate an intrapartum and a postpartum care plan and explain this to the patient.

You have 10 minutes for this task (+ 2mins initial reading time).

Instructions for Assessor

Please read the instructions for the candidate and the role player. Allow the candidate to conduct the consultation undisturbed unless they are straying off the question, in which case you should show them the instructions again.

This station is designed to test:

- Knowledge of the contemporary issues in the NHS
- Knowledge of the legal and regulatory requirements for FGM
- Communication skills

Once the candidate has taken the history and explained the Law regarding FGM, discussed the issues, outlined the care and has reached the stage of clinical examination, the candidate should ask for the examination findings. Only on request provide the following information:

- General examination—patient healthy
- Abdominal examination—uterus 16 weeks size
- Speculum examination—quite difficult as narrowing of the vagina with formation of a possible covering seal and approximation of labia minora

Should the candidate request this information prematurely gently delay the information, prompting the candidate to the instruction sheet? On divulging the examination findings, the candidate should be able to classify this as Type 3 FGM: if the candidate does not state this explicitly gentle prompting is acceptable. Now ask the candidate to explain the management plan for intrapartum and postpartum care to the patient.

There are 2 marks allocated for the role player to assign at the end of this station.

Record your overall clinical impression (Pass/Borderline/Fail) for the candidate for each of the four domains.

Instructions for Role Player

You are Mrs Arayomi Adebola, aged 30, from Somalia. You have now lived in the UK for around three years with your husband, a 34-year-old taxi driver. You have no other family members in the UK. You are a housewife. You rate your English as 'acceptable' as you can 'get by'.

You recall vividly your mum telling you that you have been 'cut down below'. You do not know any more details. You consider yourself in good general health. Otherwise you have no gynaecological or urinary or bowel complaints. You have not yet attended for a cervical smear, preferring to wait until after the childbirth. You have always found sex 'very uncomfortable', but believe this is due to the genital surgery that you have had early on and have accepted it. You are aware of the scars in the genital region.

This is your first pregnancy. You have had your routine booking bloods with your Midwife. You have informed the midwife about the 'cutting' when she took the booking history from you. You understand that this is the reason for the referral to the hospital Antenatal Clinic, although you do resent 'the fuss about what happened many years ago'.

At the hospital you are on your own. You are bewildered by the legal requirements and shocked on hearing the mention of the Police and the Social Services involvement. You however soon overcome the shock and participate in discussion as you are told that the Police involvement would not be necessary in your case.

You abhor the practice of female genital mutilation and cannot see any benefit to it. You have no intention of inflicting it on your child. Indeed you will do all that you can to protect your child from FGM. Your husband also shares the same views.

You are shocked and upset when the Doctor mentions the possibility of deinfibulation, but when pointed out that this will increase your chances of a successful vaginal delivery and long term sexual comfort, you accept it. You are relieved that this is not 'further genital surgery'.

Ideas: You are expecting an internal examination as you are aware the referral was for genital cutting. You are not expecting any operation prior to delivery.

Concerns: You are hoping that you will be able to have a normal vaginal delivery, although you anticipate that this will be difficult considering the painful sexual intercourse. You are worried that the doctor will blame you for your 'cutting'.

Expectations: You expect the doctor to explain the implications of FGM:

- The clinical implications
- The legal implications
- The impact on labour
- Any measures to improve the normal vaginal delivery rates
- Post-delivery care
- Care of the newborn

Assessment

Marking Scheme

Patient safety:

Pass Borderline Fail

Communication with patients and their relatives:

Pass Borderline Fail

Information gathering:

Pass Borderline Fail

Applied clinical knowledge:

Pass Borderline Fail

Notes for Marking

Patient safety

- Takes effort to put the patient at ease
- Involves the patient in decision making process
- Sensitively addresses legal aspects of FGM
- Adopts a no-blame approach
- Requests senior input into the assessment and management of the patient
- Negotiates a mutually agreed safe plan
- Non-judgemental approach to the patient
- Open and honest about explaining confidentiality and its limitation
- Sincere in explaining the need for referral to external agencies if the child is at risk
- Honest about the legal offences regarding FGM

Communication with patients and their relatives

- Greets patient
- Introduces self and role
- Confirms patient identity
- Assesses patient's starting point
- Explains the legal issues in simple terms, including anonymization of data
- Culturally sensitive behaviour
- Clear organized explanation in a logical sequence
- Provides information in reasonable chunks
- Allows patient time to react

- Checks patient's understanding
- Appropriate non-verbal behaviour
- Summarizes the information

Information gathering

- Obtains a relevant and sensitive history regarding the circumstances of undergoing FGM
- Obtains a relevant history about the effects of FMG

Applied clinical knowledge

- Demonstrates a sound understanding and comprehensive evidence-based Shares factually correct information with the patient
- Offers an interpreter and does not use the family member
- Aware of the legal and regulatory responsibilities
- Aware of the FGM Safeguarding Risk Assessment Tool
- Aware of the Health and Social Care Information Centre enhanced dataset
- Aware of the requirements for reporting to the Police and Social Services
- Explains to the patient the short term and the long term complications of FGM
- Communicates to the patient the need for high risk consultant-led care
- Offers a referral for psychological assessment
- Offers screening for blood borne viruses: hepatitis B, C and HIV
- Assesses for other obstetric risk factors
- Agrees and documents plan for antenatal, intrapartum, and postpartum care
- Sensitively explores the woman's own views on FGM and her plans for her children
- Takes into account the patient's family's views when formulating a care plan
- Explains to the patient intrapartum care where perineal tears are managed as for women without FGM and the high risk status for caesarean section, haemorrhage and perineal trauma
- Explains postpartum care to the patient where history of maternal FGM is recorded in the personal child health record
- If a baby girl is born, explains the process that the safeguarding midwife will notify the GP and the health visitor

Notes for Candidate

You do not need to know in detail regarding the Health and Social Care Information Centre or the FGM Safeguarding Risk Assessment Tool. You only need to know this information and how and where to access this information. You only need to explain to the patient that the Risk Assessment Tool will be done by your senior/consultant/safeguarding midwife. The assessors are aware that this is not a regular occurrence in most hospitals, although this has featured prominently in the media in the recent past.

Although you are expected to make a clinical assessment of assessment of FGM you are not required or expected to make a decision regarding deinfibulation.

Take a methodical history and assess for other high risk factors.

Further reading

Female Genital Mutilation and its Management, RCOG Green-top Guideline No. 53 July 2015. https://www.rcog.org.uk/globalassets/documents/guidelines/gtg-53-fgm.pdf

Task 3 **Antenatal screening**

Instructions for Candidate

This task assesses the following clinical skills:

- Patient safety
- Communication with patients and their relatives
- Information gathering
- Applied clinical knowledge

Michelle Taylor who is a 42-year-old teacher. She is 12 weeks pregnant and has presented to the antenatal clinic to discuss first trimester screening and its implications.

Please take a brief history and answer her questions re screening.

You have 10 minutes for this task (+ 2mins initial reading time).

Instruction for Assessor

Please read instructions to candidate and actor.

Allow the candidate to conduct the interview undisturbed unless they are straying off topic.

Record your overall clinical impression of the candidate for each domain (e.g. should this performance be pass, borderline, or a fail).

Instructions for Role Player

You are Michelle Taylor, a 42-year-old teacher, in your first ongoing pregnancy.

This is an IVF pregnancy. Two frozen embryos were transferred. This is your fourth IVF cycle. You are known to have endometriosis and have had previous key hole surgery for an ovarian cyst five years ago. You had an ectopic pregnancy following a fresh IVF cycle three years ago. You suffer from hayfever and have allergy to Penicillin.

You have had a viability scan at six weeks of gestation in the IVF clinic. You have had a vaginal bleeding at nine weeks and a scan in the early pregnancy clinic that thankfully confirmed all was well. This is a singleton ongoing pregnancy.

You were then offered a screening test in the first trimester. You are not keen to undergo any tests unless you know what the screening test involves, how accurate it is and what if it shows that your baby is at high risk to have one of the chromosomal problems. Your friend underwent a miscarriage after a needle test and the results were normal!

You have requested an appointment in the antenatal clinic to discuss the screening test. You are currently 12 weeks pregnant.

You have not had any further bleeding,

Temperament: You are very anxious about the screening test and would like to understand your options.

Ideas: You are hoping that the consultant performs a scan and tells you everything is good. You are very worried about the possibility that the screening test may indicate you are high risk because of your age.

Expectations: You want the doctor to explain the following:

- Options at this stage of pregnancy
- When can the scan be performed? Does it depend on the baby size?
- What does the scan look at and what does it indicate?

- How accurate are the results of screening?
- Who will need the needle test?
- What does the needle test involve?
- Risks associated with the procedure
- Who will be doing it?
- How accurate are the results?
- When will you get the results?
- How will you be informed of the results?
- What if you decline the invasive test?

Assessment

Marking Scheme

Patient safety:

Pass	Borderline	Fail

Communication with patients and their relatives:

Pass	Borderline	Fail

Information gathering:

Pass	Borderline	Fail

Applied clinical knowledge:

Pass	Borderline	Fail

Notes for Marking

Patient safety

- Assesses the patient's main concerns and ideas
- Discussed options for invasive testing
- Discusses risks
- Involves patient in the process (e.g. encouraging them to express their ideas, or preferences)
- Negotiates a mutually agreed acceptable, safe, plan
- Open and honest about procedure, and possible complications

Communication with patients and their relatives

- Greets, introduces self and role, checks patient's name
- Consent to proceed and explains nature of interview
- Assesses patient's starting point (what the patient wants to know) and sets the agenda
- Clear organized explanation in logical sequence
- Chunks: e.g. provides information in reasonable chunks
- Checks patient's understanding
- Language (easily understood, avoids or explains jargon)
- Uses visual aids appropriately e.g. diagrams or uses analogies to aid explanation
- Presents a clear and succinct history to the assessor

Information gathering

- Obtains a relevant obstetric history
- Obtains views on ideas, expectations, and concerns regarding screening

Applied clinical knowledge

- Gathers the relevant information in the history
- Demonstrates a sound and comprehensive evidence-based clinical knowledge for antenatal screening for Downs syndrome
- National standards for antenatal screening programme for Downs syndrome
- Trisomy 21 detection rates of 90% for a screen positive rate <2%
- Increased Nuchal translucency >/= 3.5mm increased risk of chromosomal/genetic abnormalities, cardiac defects
- NT can be performed between 11 + 2 to 14 + 1 weeks.
- The CRL should be between 45–84mm
- Different options for screening in the first and second trimester
- The combined test uses maternal age, nuchal translucency (NT) measurement and two biochemical serum markers-free β HCG and PAPP-A together with gestational age calculated from Crown Rump Length measurement
- Explaining results of screening and implications
- Detection rates and limitations of anomaly screening
- Risk of >/ = 1:150 is used as a cut off to classify as high risk
- Who should be offered invasive testing
- Risks of invasive testing of amniocentesis and chorion villous sampling 1% risk of miscarriage
- Fetal echo to be arranged with fetal medicine specialist/fetal cardiologist
- Explains options for plan of management if patient declines invasive testing

Notes for Candidate

The scenario is taken from a common clinical scenario of our daily practice. It not only assesses the process of communication but also assesses the content of the knowledge given to the patient. It is important *how* you provide the information to the patient.

Practice this scenario with one of your friends who can act as a role player and ask another friend to provide you with feedback.

Further reading

NHS Fetal Anomaly Screening Programme Screening for Down's syndrome: UK NSC Policy recommendations 2011–2014 Model of Best Practice. http://anr-dpn.vjf.cnrs.fr/sites/default/files/NSCModel-of-Best-Practice-DS%20screening2011-2014Sept2011.pdf

Amniocentesis and Chorionic Villus Sampling, Green top Guideline No 8. https://www.rcog.org.uk/globalassets/documents/guidelines/gtg_8.pdf

Task 4 **SFGA**

Instructions for Candidate

This task assesses the following clinical skills:

- Patient safety
- Communication with patients and their relatives
- Information gathering
- Applied clinical knowledge

You are an ST5 doctor in the antenatal clinic. You are asked to see Karen Grainger who is a 36-year-old lady 14 weeks into her second pregnancy. She has been referred by her midwife because her first child was born at 41 weeks by normal vaginal delivery weighing 2.9Kg which plotted <10th centile on her GROW chart. This is her first visit to the antenatal clinic. Take an appropriate history, compose an on-going management plan and answer any questions she may have.

You have 10 minutes for this task (+ 2mins initial reading time).

Instructions for Assessor

This task assesses the candidate's ability to take a focussed history and make a shared decision plan of management.

Record your overall clinical impression of the candidate for each domain (i.e. pass, borderline or fail).

There are marks for the actor to also assign at the end of the station.

Instructions for Role Player

You are Karen Grainger a 36-year-old mother of three-year-old Clara. You are currently 14 weeks pregnant. You had a previous straight forward pregnancy and delivery with Clara but were told at birth she was smaller than expected. You saw your midwife regularly throughout and were told all was measuring fine. She had some problems with feeding initially requiring a short hospital stay but was otherwise well and is developing as expected. You are healthy. You take no regular medications and have no allergies. You smoke 15 cigarettes a day, have been thinking about cutting down but are unsure what you can try in pregnancy or what support is available. You do not drink alcohol. Your dating US was normal and screening tests were low risk for Down's syndrome.

Temperament: You are anxious about doing the best for your baby but generally calm.

Ideas: You are expecting this pregnancy to be straight forward but have concerns about having another small baby. You are not sure exactly what the midwife meant by small baby as Clara seemed fine to you.

Concerns: You are concerned that Clara was felt to be small and no one picked up on this, could this happen again?

- Why was Clara so small, can this happen again? Why was this not detected?
- Can anything be done to decrease the chances of having another small baby?
- Can anything be done to detect a small baby?
- Does smoking have an effect; is there anything available to help me cut down?
- What will happen if this baby is small?

Assessment

Marking Scheme		
Patient safety:		
Pass	Borderline	Fail
Communication with patients and their relatives:		
Pass	Borderline	Fail
Information gathering:		
Pass	Borderline	Fail
Applied clinical knowledge:		
Pass	Borderline	Fail

Notes for Marking

Patient safety

- Assess patients concerns and ideas
- Respond sensitively to patients questions
- Involves patient in the process
- Agreed, acceptable safe management plan

Communication with patients and their relatives

- Greets, introduces self and role, checks patients name
- Consent to proceed and explains nature of discussion
- Sets agenda and assesses patients perception
- Organized structured approach
- Provides information in chunks
- Language (easily understood, avoids/explains jargon)

Information gathering

- Obstetric history
  - LMP, dating US, screening tests, booking bloods
  - History of current pregnancy
  - Previous obstetric history and mode of delivery (chronology, gravidity, parity)
- Personal History (past medical history, medications, allergies)
- Family History (genetics, diabetes, hypertension, thromboembolism)
- Social History (social circumstance, support network, smoking, alcohol, drugs)

Applied clinical knowledge

- Management—makes a robust and safe plan
  - Serial growth scans to assess fetal well being
  - Monitor fetal movements, attend for review if any concerns
  - Consider IOL from 37/40 if <10th Centile on ultrasound (earlier if other concerns)
  - Smoking cessation, support groups, nicotine replacement, benefits pregnancy and long-term

Notes for Candidate

Small for gestational age (SFGA) is defined as <10th centile at birth on a customized growth chart.

All women should be assessed at booking for risk factors and appropriate surveillance arranged as needed.

Risk factors are divided into:

- Major—Age >40, smoking ≥11 cigarettes/day, cocaine use, daily vigorous exercise, previous history SFGA, previous stillbirth, chronic hypertension, diabetes/vascular disease, renal impairment, APLS (Anti Phospholipid Syndrome), PET, echogenic bowel, recurrent APH, BMI <18, low PAPP-A <0.4MoM
- Minor—≥35, nulliparity, BMI <20, BMI 25–29.9, Smoking 1–10 cigarettes/day

Women with three or more minor risk factors require uterine artery doppler at 20–24 weeks if normal they should have a growth scan in the third trimester. Women with one or more major risk factor or three minor with abnormal uterine artery doppler require serial growth scans from 26–28 weeks.

Timing of delivery is guided by ultrasound assessment:

- <10th centile EFW/AC, normal umbilical doppler—ultrasound EFW/doppler fortnightly, offer delivery by 37 weeks
- <10th centile EFW/AC, EDF present but raised PI—ultrasound EFW weekly, doppler twice weekly, consider delivery by 37 weeks, sooner if static growth
- <10th centile EFW/AC, absent or reversed EDF—weekly ultrasound EFW, daily doppler or computerized CTG, recommend delivery by 32 weeks after steroids, consider 30–32 if Ductus Venosus Doppler is abnormal

Further reading

Green-top Guideline No. 31, 2nd Edition | February 2013 | Minor revisions—January 2014. https://www.rcog.org.uk/globalassets/documents/guidelines/gtg_31.pdf

Task 5 **Identifying common fetal problems–echogenic bowel**

Instructions for Candidate

This task assesses the following clinical skills:

- Patient safety
- Communication with patients and their relatives
- Information gathering
- Applied clinical knowledge

You are the ST4 and seeing Claire Smith in antenatal clinic with a scan report. Claire is 24 years old in her first pregnancy and her scan reported an echogenic bowel of the foetus at 19 weeks. Claire and her partner Thomas are here to discuss this report. The role player will ask you the following questions:

- What is it?
- What causes it?
- How common is it?
- What next?

Please gather relevant information, address her concerns and give her a plan of management for the rest of her pregnancy.

You have 10 minutes for this task (+2mins initial reading time).

Instructions for Assessor

Please read instructions to candidate and actor.

Allow the candidate to conduct the interview undisturbed unless they are straying off the track of the question (in which case you can show them their instructions again).

The candidate should start by checking pre-existing information with the patient. They should explain the scan findings in simple words avoiding medical jargons.

What is it?

This is a finding in ultrasound when the bowel of the foetus appears as bright as the bone.

What causes it?

- Usually no underlying cause is found and majority of foetuses with this isolated finding are normal.
- An association is however found with the following:
  - Chromosome anomalies such as Trisomy 21
  - Cystic Fibrosis (secondary to meconium viscosity)
  - Congenital viral infections like CMV causing inflammation of bowel mucosa
  - Intrauterine growth restriction
  - Bowel obstruction

How common is it?

This finding is seen in less than 1% of pregnancies and majority of the babies will be normal.

What next?

Any further management will depend on the cause so further testing is required to establish or rule out a cause. She will be referred to foetal medicine for a detailed scan to rule out any other associated findings. Further testing that can be offered are:

- Parental testing for CF mutation
- Maternal blood tests for CMV
- Amniocentesis for karyotyping or foetal infection

The candidate should undertake a brief discussion around each cause and check patient's pre-existing understanding on the conditions previously discussed. They should mention the option of termination in reference with CMV and Trisomy 21.

Record your overall clinical impression of the candidate for each domain (e.g. should this performance be pass, borderline, or a fail).

Instructions for Role Player

You are Claire Smith, 24 years old and this is your very first pregnancy. You were not looking forward to be pregnant and it was an 'accident', but after a while you coped with the situation and accepted the fact. Your partner is Thomas Edward, 32 years old, and is in good health. Both of you are Caucasians. You had your routine anomaly scan at 19 weeks after which you were referred to antenatal clinic to discuss the report with the doctor.

You should ask the following questions from the candidate?

- What is it?
- What causes it?
- How common is it?
- What next?

Temperament: You are very worried with this scan report and wonder if you have done something in very early pregnancy that might have resulted in this abnormal finding. Although you were not prepared for this pregnancy, you never considered a termination.

Ideas: You have no idea of what this finding means. You have an understanding of a condition called Cystic Fibrosis because one of your cousins has the disease.

Concerns: You are concerned if this is due to an unplanned pregnancy. You are also concerned if this can result in a serious damage to your baby.

Expectations: You would like to have a clear understanding of what this condition is and what it might mean. You would also like to know if this can cause any abnormality or death of your baby. You can consider a termination if any serious effects on baby are expected.

Assessment

Marking Scheme

Patient safety:

Pass Borderline Fail

Communication with patients and their relatives:

Pass Borderline Fail

Information gathering:
Pass Borderline Fail

Applied clinical knowledge:
Pass Borderline Fail

Notes for Marking

Patient safety

- Assesses the patient's main concerns and ideas. Refers to the fetial medicine for further follow-up. Offers information leaflets
- Open and honest about amniocentesis and possible complications. Provides with information about the person performing the procedure and safeguard in place e.g. competent clinician or junior doctor under direct supervision
- Explains mechanisms in place to deal with complications

Communication with patients and their relatives

- Greets, introduces self and role, checks patient's name
- Consent to proceed and explains nature of interview
- Assesses patient's starting point (what the patient wants to know) and sets the agenda
- Clear organized explanation in logical sequence
- Chunks: i.e. provides information in reasonable chunks
- Checks patient's understanding.
- Language (easily understood, avoids or explains jargon)
- Uses visual aids appropriately e.g. diagrams or uses analogies to aid explanation

Information gathering

- Obtains a relevant obstetric history
- Obtains views, ideas, expectations, and concerns regarding Cystic Fibrosis

Applied clinical knowledge

- Demonstrates a sound and comprehensive evidence-based clinical knowledge of the condition and its implications. Addresses each cause individually and explains to the patient. Provides a clear follow-up plan. Also mentions the risks associated with invasive procedures like amniocentesis

Notes for Candidate

The scenario is taken from a common clinical scenario of our daily practice. It not only assesses the process of communication but also assesses the content of the knowledge given to the patient. It is important how you provide the information to the patient.

Practice this scenario with one of your friends who can act as a role player and ask another friend to provide you with feedback.

Further reading

NHS screening patient information leaflet, http://www.fetalanomaly.screening.nhs.uk/
Cystic Fibrosis. http://www.cysticfibrosis.org.uk/

Task 6 **Identifying maternal health problems**

Instructions to Candidate

This task assesses the following clinical skills:

- Patient safety
- Communication with patients and their relatives
- Information gathering
- Applied clinical knowledge

You are an ST5 doctor working in the maternity day unit. You are asked to see Priya Patel.

She is a primip who is 32 weeks pregnant with a singleton pregnancy.

She has been suffering with itching symptoms for the last couple of weeks. The midwife in the day unit has ordered some blood tests.

Please take a brief history and look at the results provided, in order to make a diagnosis and a management plan.

Your task is to:

- Make a diagnosis
- Formulate an appropriate management plan
- Justify your answers

Blood results

Hb—115
WCC—5.4
PLTS—156
Na—137
K—3.6
Urea—2.6
Creat—60
Alk phos—35
ALT—70
AST—40
Albumin—18
Bile acids—13

You have 10 minutes for this task (+ 2mins initial reading time).

Instructions for Assessor

Please read instruction to candidate and actor.

Allow the candidate to conduct the interview undisturbed unless they are straying off the track of the question (in which case you can show them their instructions again).

Record your overall clinical impression of the candidate for each domains (i.e. should this performance be pass, borderline, or a fail).

Instruction for Role Player

You are Priya Patel, a 25-year-old who is 32 weeks pregnant with her first child.

You have had an uneventful pregnancy so far, but have developed some itching in the last couple of weeks. You have noticed that it is particularly bad on the palms of your hand and soles of your feet. Your GP gave you some Piriton tablet, which has helped a bit, but you still find it hard to sleep as it's particularly bad at night. You remember that your sister had a lot of itching in her pregnancy too.

Your baby has been moving well, but you are concerned that your bump isn't as big as some of the others in your antenatal class.

When you are given the diagnosis of obstetric cholestasis, you want to know:

- What are the treatment options, can it be cured?
- What impact it will have on your baby, what are the associated risks and complications?
- Will it affect how you can deliver the baby?
- Will you need extra monitoring?
- Will it affect your health in the long term?
- Will it affect future pregnancies?
- Why has it happened?

Assessment

Marking Scheme

Patient safety:

Pass	Borderline	Fail

Communication with patients and their relatives:

Pass	Borderline	Fail

Information gathering:

Pass	Borderline	Fail

Applied clinical knowledge:

Pass	Borderline	Fail

Notes for Marking

Patient safety

- Assesses the patient's main concerns and ideas
- Gives options and discusses the pros and cons of different management plans
- Discusses possible complications and measures to reduce them
- Involves patient in the process (e.g. encouraging them to express their ideas, or preferences)
- Negotiates a mutually agreed acceptable, safe, plan
- Open and honest about procedure and possible complications
- Provides patient with information about the person performing the procedure and safeguard in place i.e. competent clinician or junior doctor under direct supervision. Explains mechanism in

place to deal with complications and learn from complications. Is honest about prolongation of recovery time if untoward complication happen

Communication with patients and their relatives

- Greets, introduces self and role, checks patient's name
- Consent to proceed and explains nature of interview
- Assesses patient's starting point (what the patient wants to know) and sets the agenda
- Clear organized explanation in logical sequence
- Chunks: i.e. provides information in reasonable chunks
- Checks patient's understanding.
- Language (easily understood, avoids or explains jargon)
- Uses visual aids appropriately e.g. diagrams or uses analogies to aid explanation
- Presents a clear and succinct management plan to the assessor

Information gathering

- Obtains a relevant obstetric history
- Obtains views, ideas, expectations, and concerns regarding this condition

Applied clinical knowledge

- Demonstrates a sound and comprehensive evidence-based clinical knowledge
- This patient has obstetric cholestasis and the management should include:
- Explanation of diagnosis—derangement of liver function and build up of bile acids
- Possible genetic component
- Typical symptoms are itching, occasionally jaundice
- Effects on baby—increased chance of meconium being passed; increased chance of premature delivery; possible increased risk of still birth
- Bloods and ultrasound to rule out other causes
- No cure except delivery
- Piriton, lotions, UDCA, consider vit. K
- Monitoring of bloods
- Induction of labour after 37 weeks
- Increased chance of recurrence in subsequent pregnancies

Further reading

Green top guideline, No 43, 2011. https://www.rcog.org.uk/globalassets/documents/guidelines/gtg_43.pdf

Chapter 10 **Maternal medicine**

Task 1 **Diabetes**

Instructions for Candidates

This task assesses the following clinical skills:

- Patient safety
- Communication with patients and their relatives
- Information gathering
- Applied clinical knowledge

You are an ST5 doctor in the diabetic antenatal clinic. The clinic has been particularly busy today and is running 60 minutes late. There are several different clinics running simultaneously and no extra staff available to help in the diabetic clinic. You are asked to see Claire Potter, a 28-year-old lady with Type 1 diabetes who is 32 weeks in her first pregnancy. She has no other medical risk factors and her diabetes is well controlled with no complications. A recent HBA1c was 45. Ultrasound today shows normal liquor and normal symmetrical growth plotting on her established growth curve at 75th centile.

Conduct a focused antenatal review and respond to her concerns.

You have 10 minutes for this task (+ 2mins initial reading time).

Instructions for Assessor

This task assesses the communication skills and application of knowledge regarding diabetes in pregnancy.

Please do not interrupt or prompt.

Record your overall clinical impression of the candidate for each domain (i.e. pass, borderline, or fail).

There are marks for the actor to also assign at the end of the station

Instruction for Role Player

You are Claire Potter, a 28-year-old solicitor, 32 weeks into your first pregnancy. You have Type 1 diabetes since you were 12 and are very confident in how best to control your diabetes. You are meticulous with checking your BM's and adjusting your insulin accordingly and they are all within range (4–6.5).

You have no complications of diabetes and no other health problems. You take short and long acting insulin and have no allergies. You do not smoke or drink alcohol. You're dating and anomaly ultrasound scans were normal and screening tests were low risk for Down's syndrome. Your pregnancy has been uneventful with regular clinic reviews of your diabetes. Your last scan at 28/40 showed the baby was growing normally.

Temperament: You are a very busy professional person and do not like to be kept waiting unnecessarily. You are annoyed the clinic is running late (yet again) but are not unreasonable provided you feel you are being listened to and your concerns addressed. You intend to raise your concerns with the doctor at the start of the consultation. You like to be informed of your management and take an active role in decision making.

Ideas: You are annoyed the clinic is running late again and that it appears patients who arrived after you are being seen first. You also don't feel that the doctor you saw last time addressed your questions regarding timing of delivery and was quite dismissive. You are keen for a vaginal birth if possible.

Concerns: You are concerned that you have been delayed because your notes have been mislaid and that is why someone else has been seen first. When you asked the receptionist she was unable to tell you how long the wait was or when you would be seen. You are concerned the doctor will be dismissive of your questions again like last time. You want to know when you will be delivered so that you can plan your work schedule and maternity leave accordingly. Your partner works away frequently so you need as much notice as possible as you really want him to be present at the birth. You wish to raise your concerns regarding the previous doctor's attitude being unacceptable.

You also want to find out the following:

- Why is the clinic running so late? Why have other people been seen first who arrived after you?
- Is everything ok with the ultrasound scan?

Assessment

Patient safety:
Pass Borderline Fail

Communication with patients and their relatives:
Pass Borderline Fail

Information gathering:
Pass Borderline Fail

Applied clinical knowledge:
Pass Borderline Fail

Notes for Marking

Patient safety

- Assess patients concerns and ideas
- Respond sensitively to patients questions
- Involves patient in the process
- Agreed, acceptable safe management plan
- Open and honest about the reasons of delay in the clinic
- Offers apology for delay
- Explains multiple clinics and other patients may be seeing different doctors and that her notes have not been mislaid
- Offers apology that she felt last doctor was dismissive of her concerns but do not incriminate colleague
- Fully discuss concerns today and ensure patient feels listened to
- Explain will feedback her concerns to consultants/management that clinic frequently runs late to assess if improvements can be made to reduce delays

- Suggest clinic staff have a noticeboard which is kept up to date of clinic delays in waiting area
- Audit clinic waiting times
- Complaints procedure, offer PALS

Communication with patients and their relatives

- Greets, introduces self and role, checks patients name
- Consent to proceed and explains nature of discussion
- Allows patient time to express concerns without interrupting
- Maintains eye contact, open posture
- Sets agenda and assesses patients perception
- Organized structured approach
- Provides information in chunks

Information gathering

- Obstetric History
  - LMP, dating US, anomaly US, screening results
  - History of current pregnancy (foetal movements, BP/urine, new symptoms)
  - Diabetes (BM's, current treatment, enquire about any hypoglycaemia)
- Diabetes History (duration, management, complications, renal/retinal screening, check has glucagon or equivalent, driving rules)
- Social History (social circumstance, support network, smoking, alcohol, drugs)

Applied clinical knowledge

- Explain ultrasound findings (normal growth)
- Management—makes a robust and safe plan
  - Serial growth scans to assess foetal well-being (next 34–36 weeks)
  - Monitor foetal movements, attend for review if any concerns
  - Recommend delivery from 38 weeks likely IOL (unless concerns sooner)
  - Importance of informing if concerns with hyper or hypoglycaemia and numbers to contact
  - MDT input from diabetic team/dietician
  - Arrange appropriate follow up in two weeks

Notes for Candidate

Good blood glucose control in the prenatal and antenatal period reduces the risk of miscarriage, congenital malformations, stillbirth and neonatal death. The aim is to optimize glucose control which requires increased monitoring throughout pregnancy.

Women should be managed in a joint obstetric-diabetic clinic. Patients should be monitored preconceptually and antenatally for signs of complications—retinal screening, renal dysfunction and hypertension. They should also have an HBA1c each trimester.

All women should be recommended to take high dose folic acid (5mg) and low dose aspirin from 12 weeks unless contraindicated.

Pregnancy places an increasing insulin demand so women with Type 1 diabetes will require increasing insulin doses as the pregnancy progresses. This demand falls postnatally when doses need to be reduced and risk of hypoglycaemia increases.

There is an increased risk of hypoglycaemia with tight control, particularly in the first trimester often associated with hyperemesis so it is important they are aware of this and have immediate access to glucose solutions or glucagon.

All patients with diabetes require serial scans to assess for signs of macrosomia, polyhydramnios or indications for early delivery.

The NICE guideline recommends delivery at 37–38 + 6 weeks for women with pre-existing diabetes. Women should be aware of the increased risk of shoulder dystocia.

Further reading

Diabetes in pregnancy: management from preconception to the postnatal period: NICE guideline [NG3] Published date: February 2015 last updated: August 2015. https://www.nice.org.uk/guidance/ng3?unlid=2068841242016109211840

Task 2 **Infectious disease**

Instructions for Candidate

This task assesses the following clinical skills:

- Patient safety
- Communication with colleagues
- Information gathering
- Applied clinical knowledge

You are the ST4 on call and receive a phone call from the community midwife who is seeing a lady who is currently 12 weeks pregnant and her son has developed chicken pox. The same midwife calls you again after 48 hours and a week later with new information, asking your advice.

Please gather relevant information and provide her with a plan of management on each of the three situations.

You have 10 minutes for this task (+ 2mins initial reading time).

Instructions for Assessor

Please read instructions to candidate and actor.

Allow the candidate to conduct the interview undisturbed unless they are straying off the track of the question (in which case you can show them their instructions again).

Record your overall clinical impression of the candidate for each domain (e.g. should this performance be pass, borderline, or a fail).

Instructions for Role Player

You are a community midwife and you will call the obstetrician on three occasions with information regarding the same patient. The patient you are seeing is Mrs. Angel Smith, 12 weeks pregnant and her son developed a rash that is suspected to be chicken pox. On the first call, you called the obstetrician to take their advice in this regards. The obstetrician will ask you some questions related to history of Angel and you will provide them with the following information:

The rash on her three-year-old child has appeared two days ago, and some vesicles are now starting to appear. Angel doesn't think she has ever had chicken pox. Her mother is not alive and she can't confirm this information. On this occasion the candidate will ask you to request some tests for Angel, called VZ IgG. If they don't give you any follow-up instructions on this test results, prompt them and ask what to do with the results. If the results are positive for IgG, you will be told to reassure the patient that she is immune for chicken pox and requires no further treatment. They also tell you that if the result is negative, she will require further treatment.

You, however, call them back in 48 hours with the results, which came out to be negative. The candidate should tell you that in this case she needs the immunoglobulin injection. Ask the candidate if the time frame to give this injection is fine. If they do not themselves offer a follow-up advice, prompt them and ask if there is any information that needs to be given to the patient. Also ask about their follow-up plan and if any extra surveillance of her pregnancy is required after the immunoglobulin.

Angela receives the injection but still develops mild chicken pox infection. However, according to the previously given follow-up advice, she contacted her GP and has received acyclovir. She is not very worried about her symptoms, but she is concerned about effects of this infection and the medications on her pregnancy. So you make a third call to the doctor to seek their advice on this.

Temperament: You are an extra cautious midwife and want to check everything with the doctor before advising to the patient.

Ideas: You are already aware of all the steps to be taken at all three levels of consultation but are more keen on having a clear management and follow-up plan that you can document.

Concerns: You forward concerns raised by the patient with regards to effects of chicken pox on the unborn and then you want to know if this woman requires a hospital referral, or can still carry on follow-up with you and her GP.

Expectations: On every phone call, you expect the doctor to take patient's history from you, provide you a clear management of the presenting problems and a clear follow-up plan, as well as advice to be given to Angela.

Assessment

Marking Scheme

Patient safety:

Pass	Borderline	Fail

Communication with colleagues:

Pass	Borderline	Fail

Information gathering:

Pass	Borderline	Fail

Applied clinical knowledge:

Pass	Borderline	Fail

Notes for Marking

Patient safety

- Assesses the patient's main concerns and ideas on every stage and addresses them appropriately as mentioned above
- Being honest about acyclovir

Communication with colleague

- Clear and concise
- Non-patronising and professional

Information gathering

- Obtains relevant information about the patient from the community midwife

Applied clinical knowledge

Demonstrates a sound and comprehensive evidence-based clinical knowledge for every stage of the scenario. Addresses present situation and gives a clear follow-up. The candidate should start by taking relevant history on each occasion. This should cover the following points:

Telephone Call 1:

- Identifies significant exposure by asking the age of the child who developed rash.
- Timing of exposure.
- Type of rash and if it is confirmed as varicella Zoster virus infection.
- Check immunity status of the patient.

Telephone Call 2:

- Recall on previous history and confirms if the exposure is within ten days.

Telephone Call 3:

- Confirms the severity of symptoms, type of rash, associated symptoms.
- Confirms her treatment history.

After taking history in each call, the candidate should be able to provide relevant advice on the present situation, as well as a follow-up plan on that advice:

Telephone Call 1:

- Check her blood serology for VZV IgG.
- If positive for IgG, she can be reassured and no further treatment is needed. (Up to 90% of women are immune).
- If negative for IgG, she should be advised to receive IgG at the earliest. If administered within ten days of exposure, it is thought to prevent chicken pox developing or reduce the severity of any infection.

Telephone Call 2:

- She should be advised to receive VZV IgG. Confirm she has no symptoms herself. Confirm the stage of her child's symptoms.
- The woman should be advised that if she develops a rash after the injection, she should contact her GP immediately and stay away from other pregnant women and neonates, until the lesions have crusted over.
- Symptomatic treatment and advice on hygiene to avoid secondary infection.
- She may be considered to be started on Acyclovir (800mg five times a day) if the rash develops within 24 hours of the immunoglobulin. This can reduce the length of the symptoms of chicken pox. Although, use below 20 weeks should be with caution and may be considered based on severity of symptoms. Patient should be informed that Acyclovir is not licensed for use in pregnancy and data on its association with foetal malformations is inconclusive.
- She should also be warned that if she develops any respiratory symptoms or deteriorates following development of the rash she should attend the hospital.

Telephone Call 3:

- Reassure this doesn't increase the risk of miscarriage; however there is a small risk of FVS (Fetal Varicella Syndrome). (can complicate a pregnancy between three and 28 weeks)
- She should be referred to foetal medicine unit at 16–20 weeks or five weeks after infection, for discussion and detailed ultrasound examination.
- Amniocentesis, risks vs benefits. Diagnostic for foetal infection.

Notes for Candidate

The scenario is taken from a common clinical scenario of our daily practice. It not only assesses the process of communication but also assesses the content of the knowledge given to the patient. It is important how you provide the information to the patient.

Practice this scenario with one of your friends who can act as a role player and ask another friend to provide you with feedback.

Further reading

Chicken pox in Pregnancy; Green Top Guideline Number 13, January 2015 https://www.rcog.org.uk/globalassets/documents/guidelines/gtg13.pdf

Task 3 **Thalassaemia**

Instructions for Candidate

This task assesses the following clinical skills:

- Patient safety
- Communication with patients and their relatives
- Information gathering
- Applied clinical knowledge

Instructions for Candidate

You are a ST5 doctor in the pre-conception counselling clinic. You are asked to see Saima Hussain, who is a 24-year-old lady of Pakistani origin. She is a British citizen and can communicate very well in English. She has attended for pre-conception counselling with her husband Ahmed. She was diagnosed with beta Thalassaemia intermedia during her late teenage years for which she has needed transfusions on couple of occasions. She is reasonably stable and maintains her haemoglobin around 90–95gm/l. The couple is contemplating a family and very keen to have some information regarding the risks to her and the baby. They have been referred for pre-conception counselling by their GP who is very concerned about the risks in pregnancy.

After the initial counselling, you will be provided with further information and investigation results by the examiner.

You have 10 minutes for this task (+ 2mins initial reading time).

Instruction for Assessor

Please read instruction to candidate and role player.

After initial pre-conception counselling consultation (or in the last five mins) tell the candidate that Mrs. Hussain is now pregnant and has attended the antenatal clinic at eight weeks of pregnancy. She has undergone a full assessment by the multidisciplinary joint obstetric haematology team. There was no indication for pre-pregnancy chelation. She has conceived with ovulation induction. She has been taking Folic acid (5mg) and Vitamin D supplements for the last six months.

Her pre-conception investigations are as follows:

Genetic testing of husband—not thalassemia carrier
Haemoglobin 90g/l
Glucose tolerance test and HbA1C normal
Thyroid function tests normal
Echocardiogram, electrocardiogram, cardiac MRI within acceptable range.
Liver iron <7mg/g (dry weight)
Hepatitis B and C screening negative
Ultrasound liver and gall bladder—normal

Ask the candidate to explain the care in the antenatal, intrapartum and postnatal period explaining the possible risks and complications.

Instructions for Role Player

You are Saima Hussain, 24-year-old woman, married to Ahmed. Your parents are originally from Pakistan but you are a British citizen, was born and brought up in Britain. You work as a receptionist and you husband is a store manager. You were diagnosed with beta thalassemia intermedia at the age of 17 years. This has not caused you many problems other than being anaemic. You have needed transfusions on couple of occasions and maintained haemoglobin of around 90–95gm/dl. You are otherwise stable and determined to lead a normal life. You have no other medical problems. Your husband is very supportive. You have never been pregnant before and your periods are more or less regular. You have been using combined oral contraceptive pills for contraception. Both you and Ahmed are now seriously thinking of having a baby but your GP has said that this can lead to complications for you and the baby. This has obviously made you anxious for which you wished to consult a specialist. Your GP has referred you and your husband to the hospital for a consultation with the doctors to discuss this further. Ahmed has never been tested for thalassemia but is otherwise fit and well.

Temperament: You think you are mostly a calm, level headed sensible woman, but you like to be organised, well informed with a definite plan.

Ideas: You would like to have a baby but will consider all the risks seriously. You are happy to consider other options if pregnancy is too risky.

Concerns: You are concerned about the risk of the baby having the disease. You are also concerned about your own health risks and the outcome.

Expectations: You want the doctor to explain:

- How serious is your thalassemia?
- Can you get pregnant?
- What are the additional risks to you in pregnancy?
- What are the risks to baby?
- What is the chance of baby having the disease?
- What can you do to prepare for pregnancy?
- Is there anything, which can reduce your risks of complication in the pregnancy?
- Will you need transfusions in pregnancy?
- Can you have a normal delivery?
- What happens if there is a complication?

Assessment

Marking Scheme

Patient safety:
Pass Borderline Fail

Communication with patients and their relatives:
Pass Borderline Fail

Information gathering:
Pass Borderline Fail

Applied clinical knowledge:
Pass Borderline Fail

Notes for Marking

Patient safety

- Assesses patients main concerns and ideas
- Gives options and discusses the pros and cons of each
- Involves patient in the process (encourages them to express their ideas or preferences)
- Explains need for multidisciplinary specialist input and pre-conception assessment
- Negotiates a mutually agreed, acceptable and safe management plan
- Open and honest
- Give detailed and straight forward explanation of the risks to the mother her baby
- Explain fully why complications can happen and what can be done to reduce the risks and possible complications
- Ensures that proper guideline will be followed with involvement of the multidisciplinary specialist team to offer safe and optimum management

Communication with patients and their relatives

- Greets, introduces self and role, checks patient's name
- Consent to proceed and explains nature of the interview
- Assesses what patient wants to know (starting point) and sets the agenda
- Clear organized explanation in logical sequence
- Chunks: i.e. provides information in reasonable chunks
- Checks patients understanding
- Language (easily understood, avoids or explains jargon)

Information gathering

- Obtains a relevant and focussed obstetric and medical history
- Obtains patients views, ideas, expectations, and concerns regarding Thalassemia

Aplied clinical knowledge

- Demonstrates a sound and comprehensive evidence based comprehensive knowledge
- Counsels the patient with relevant information that is factually correct
- Makes a robust and safe management plan taking patient's views into account

Notes for Candidate

Pre-conception counselling

- Take a detailed history to determine degree of the disease and whether needs transfusion
- Review medications if any
- Explain sometime can have difficulty in conceiving and may require ovulation induction
- Will need multidisciplinary input to assess multi organ status and safety, prior to pregnancy
- Partner genetic testing will be required
- Higher risk of miscarriage
- Need to exclude diabetes and thyroid disease
- Need to assess cardiac and liver status for iron overload
- Blood group and presence of red cell antibodies need to be checked.

- Will need higher dose of Folic acid and Vitamin D supplementation
- Should have screening for Hepatitis B and C
- May need chelation pre- conception if high iron load is detected.
- May need transfusions during pregnancy if haemoglobin < 80gm/l
- Risk of fatal Intrauterine growth retardation
- May need early delivery if indicated

Antenatal

- Will need multidisciplinary management and strict vigilance
- Blood pressure measurement and urine for culture sensitivity to be sent at booking
- Monthly review until 28 weeks and fortnightly thereafter will be undertaken
- Early scan seven to nine weeks to confirm viability
- Detailed scan 18–20 weeks
- 4 weekly growth scans from 24 weeks, as there is risk of foetal growth restriction
- Specialist cardiac assessment at 28 weeks and as appropriate thereafter
- May need further blood transfusion
- Transfusion can be avoided if haemoglobin above 80gm/l at 36 weeks
- Anaesthetic appointment may have to be arranged at 36 weeks if indicated
- May need postnatal blood transfusion

Labour

- Timing of delivery in line with national guidelines
- Thalassaemia is not an indication for caesarean section
- Multidisciplinary team to be involved as soon as she is admitted to labour suite
- Group and save in labour if haemoglobin level stable, otherwise will need cross match
- Continuous intrapartum foetal monitoring to determine foetal well being
- Active management of third stage to reduce bleeding

Postnatal

- Postnatal prophylactic anticoagulation to be considered as high risk of venous thromboembolism
- Breast feeding safe and should be encouraged

Further reading

Management of Beta Thalassaemia in Pregnancy Green-top Guideline No.66.RCOG March 2014. https://www.rcog.org.uk/globalassets/documents/guidelines/gtg_66_thalassaemia.pdf

Task 4 **Pre-eclampsia**

Instructions for Candidate

This task assesses the following clinical skills:

- Patient safety
- Communication with patients and their relatives
- Information gathering
- Applied clinical knowledge

You are a ST5 doctor in the antenatal clinic. You are asked to see Pamela Jones who is a 31-year-old lady in her second pregnancy. She has been referred by her midwife with previous history of pre-eclampsia. She is now 12 weeks pregnant. She had a normal vaginal delivery two years ago when she was induced at 35 weeks. She is otherwise fit and well. Dating ultrasound scan confirms singleton pregnancy 11 weeks of gestation.

Once you have finished the initial discussion with Pamela, the assessor will ask you some questions.

You have 10 minutes for this task (+ 2mins initial reading time).

Instruction for Assessor

Please read the instruction to candidate and actor

After consultation with the actor patient (or last six mins), tell the candidate that Pamela had an intrauterine foetal death (IUFD) at 37 weeks. She was referred to ANC at 35 weeks with pelvic girdle pain when her BP was 130/86 with a trace of protein. She was reassured and planned for CMW to review in one week. Her urinalysis at 36 weeks showed 2+ protein which was not actioned (told could be due to vaginal discharge) and a BP of 130/90 with the CMW. Then she is referred at 37 weeks by CMW with BP 160/109 with 2 + protein in urine sample when no foetal heart is found. IUFD is confirmed on USS.

Ask the candidate to explain the situation to Pamela. Was this preventable?

There are some marks on the process mark sheet for the actor to assign at the end of the station. Record your overall clinical impression of the candidate for each domain i.e. should this performance be a pass, borderline, of fail.

Instructions for Role Player

You are Pamela Jones, a 31-year-old mother of your two-year-old son Jack. Your pregnancy last time was complicated by pre-eclampsia for which you had to be started off (induced) at 35 weeks. The condition started developing around 29–30 weeks of gestation. You had protein in your water sample and your blood pressure (BP) was raised. You did need some tablets to control your BP. However, the blood results became abnormal and the baby stopped growing, when they made a decision for induction. You had a straight forward labour and a normal vaginal delivery. You stopped the medication for BP four weeks after delivery.

Your midwife this time has told you that this can happen again which you were not aware of. You do not understand the condition very well and is worried of this happening again.

You are otherwise fit and healthy school teacher. You live with Jack and your husband James who is a solicitor. James is father of Jack as well. You do not smoke and have not had any alcohol in pregnancy.

Temperament: You think you are mostly a clam, rational and sensible woman but like to be aware of possibilities and be in control.

Ideas: You were expecting that this pregnancy would be uncomplicated and easy being the second one, having been in and out of hospital with pre-eclampsia last time.

Concerns: You are now concerned of developing pre-eclampsia again and worried about the consequences. You also think it might be worse than last time. You are keen to know if anything can be done to prevent this happening again.

Expectations: You want the doctor to explain:

- What is pre-eclampsia?
- What is the chance of it happening again?
- Can anything be done to prevent it happening?
- How can it affect you and the baby?
- Will you have to be delivered early again?
- How will you know that you are developing pre-eclampsia?

You had an uneventful pregnancy *this time* until 35 weeks when you were referred to the antenatal clinic (ANC) with pelvic girdle pain. In ANC your BP was found to be 130/86 with a trace of protein in your urine sample. You were reassured and sent home with a plan to be followed up by the community midwife (CMW) in a week's time. At the appointment with CMW, your BP was 130/90 and urine sample showed 2 + protein. You were reassured with regards to the BP and told that the protein in the urine sample can be because of the vaginal discharge you have had. The plan was to review your BP and the urine sample in a week's time (37 weeks). At the next appointment, the CMW referred you to the hospital with a BP of 160/109 and the urinalysis showed 3 + protein. On admission to hospital, the baby's heart beat could not be detected and an intrauterine foetal death (IUFD) is confirmed following an ultrasound scan (USS).

You are devastated and angry. You want an explanation now as to why the pre-eclampsia was not picked up earlier despite having protein in urine sample and why this has happened.

You ask these questions once the assessor has provided the candidate with the information of the foetal death.

At the end there are some marks for you to award according to how well the candidate has explained your questions and concerns.

Assessment

Marking Scheme

Patient safety:

Pass	Borderline	Fail

Communication with patients and their relatives:

Pass	Borderline	Fail

Information gathering:

Pass	Borderline	Fail

Applied clinical knowledge:

Pass	Borderline	Fail

Notes for Marking

Patient safety

- Assesses patients main concerns and ideas
- Discusses effects on mother and baby
- Gives information on symptoms to be aware of and when to contact hospital
- Involves patient in the process
- Makes a safe management plan
- Open and honest
- Offer apology and condolences
- Fully explain what has happened
- Takes responsibility—pre-eclampsia can be possible cause of IUFD
- Further investigations might give more information
- Reassures process is in place to investigate the incident and action will be taken

Communication with patients and their relatives

- Greets, introduces self and role, checks patient's name
- Consent to proceed and explains nature of the interview
- Assesses patient's starting point (what patient wants to know) and sets the agenda
- Clear organized explanation in logical sequence
- Chunk: i.e. provides information in reasonable chunks
- Checks patient's understanding
- Uses analogies appropriately or to aid explanation

Information gathering

- Obtains a relevant and focussed obstetric history
- Obtains patients views, ideas, expectations, and concerns regarding pre-eclampsia

Applied clinical knowledge

- Demonstrates sound and comprehensive evidence-based clinical knowledge
- Counsels the patient with relevant information that is factually correct
- Makes a robust and safe management plan e.g. criteria for referral to the ANC

Notes for Candidate

History

- Obtain details of previous pregnancy, complications and outcome
- Degree of pre-eclampsia in previous pregnancy and reason for induction
- To ascertain cause for concern and anxiety

Explanation of pre-eclampsia

- Nature of the condition
- Risk of recurrence
- Can cause multisystem disorder in mother and foetal growth restriction due to placental insufficiency

- Sometimes can develop HELLP syndrome or eclampsia
- Depending on course of the disease, may need early delivery—risk of prematurity
- Delivery is the treatment for the condition

Management plan in this pregnancy

- To start Aspirin as per NICE recommendations for prevention
- Vigilance regarding BP and proteinuria
- Cut off BP for referral from community to maternity assessment unit
- Symptom complex to prompt referral—headache/visual disturbances/abdominal pain
- If diagnosed with pre-eclampsia, may need admission, BP monitoring, treatment for BP, Protein-creatinine ratio, 24 hours protein, obstetric ultrasound scan for foetal growth

Counselling

- Acknowledge reason for her anger
- Accept that appropriate action has not been taken
- Admit that different action could have changed the outcome
- Postmortem and other tests may help in determining cause of foetal death.
- Process of investigation and action plan to avoid this happening in future
- Duty of candour
- Will have a consultant postnatal debriefing with investigation reports.

Further reading

Hypertension in pregnancy: diagnosis and management Clinical guideline [CG107] Published date: August 2010 last updated: January 2011. https://www.nice.org.uk/guidance/cg107

Task 5 **Hypertension**

Instructions for Candidate

This task assesses the following clinical skills:

- Patient safety
- Communication with colleagues
- Information gathering
- Applied clinical knowledge

This is a discussion station with the examiner. An outline of the scenario is given. During the discussion, this scenario will evolve and the examiner will give you further details. Your discussion should be supported by evidence-based practice.

Mrs Bergman is a 29-year-old second gravida attends your antenatal clinic at 11 weeks of gestation following her dating scan. In her past pregnancy she had suffered pre-eclampsia which necessitated a delivery by caesarean section at 32 weeks of gestation. The new born male child weighed 1390 grams and is now three years of age. She is currently normotensive and has no health problems.

You have 10 minutes for this task (+ 2mins initial reading time).

Instructions for Assessor

After ensuring they have read and understood the scenario, start the discussion by asking this following questions:

- She wants to find out possible outcome of this pregnancy, how will you plan her antenatal care and management in the current pregnancy?
- What information would you like to seek from this very anxious and worried lady?
- Mrs Bergman's health has remained fine when she visits your clinic after mid trimester scan. Would you like to add anything at this point?
- At 26 weeks of gestation the community midwife referred Mrs Bergman to the antenatal day assessment unit in your department because of high blood pressure of 156/102 and proteinuria of 1^{+} on dipstick test. How will you manage her?

Record your overall clinical impression of the candidate for each domain (e.g. should this performance be pass, borderline, or a fail).

Assessment

Marking Scheme

Patient safety:

Pass Borderline Fail

Communication with colleagues:

Pass Borderline Fail

Information gathering:

Pass Borderline Fail

Applied clinical knowledge:

Pass Borderline Fail

Notes for Marking

Patient safety

- Careful patient selection
- Provides patient with information leaflets on frequent and serious risks associated with severe preeclampsia
- Mentions the importance of meticulous documentation on each occasion i.e. clinic notes, plan of care, record of information provided to the patient and follow-up plans
- Involving the consultant and discussing the case in departmental meetings.
- Shows understanding of what not to be used in treatment
- Provides with information to the patient and be honest about the risk of recurrent pre-eclampsia and preterm birth
- Explain mechanism in place to deal with complications
- Being honest about further investigations, repeat hospital admission, need for Multidisciplinary team (MDT) and an early delivery depending on the clinical situation

Communication with the colleagues

- Clear and concise communication
- Demonstrates awareness, understanding and importance of shared decision making. Shows understanding of the principles of multidisciplinary care and involves the right multidisciplinary care team member according the clinical situation

Information gathering

- Aware of the focused and relevant information that needs to be obtained from this patient

Applied clinical knowledge

- Demonstrates a sound and comprehensive evidence-based clinical knowledge—uses the reference of NICE guidance on hypertension in pregnancy to define mild, moderate and severe hypertension. Shows familiarity with the different management pathways based on these definitions
- She wants to find out possible outcome of this pregnancy, how will you plan her antenatal care and management in the current pregnancy?
- The candidate should include all or most of the following points:
    - Finds out details of previous pregnancy, onset and severity of pre-eclampsia, management of pre-eclampsia, indication and type of caesarean section, any surgical complications, puerperal recovery, and course of newborn care and how her baby is doing
- What information would you like to seek from this very anxious and worried lady?
- Medication family history of pre-eclampsia
- About a one in four chance of recurrence of pre-eclampsia
- Check BP and test urine by automated reagent strip reader
- 75mg aspirin from 12 weeks until birth (recognizes >one moderate risk factors)
- Makes a plan of care: review by community midwife every week, review in consultant Antenatal Clinic (ANC) after the routine 20-week anomaly scan (to ensure placenta is normally located and foetus is healthy)
- Mrs Bergman's health has remained fine when she visits your clinic after mid trimester scan. Would you like to add anything at this point?
- Continue same care as described

- At 26 weeks of gestation the community midwife referred Mrs Bergman to the antenatal day assessment unit in your department because of high blood pressure of 156/102 and proteinuria of 1^+ on dipstick test. How will you manage her?
- Confirms BP reading and defines as moderate hypertension (150/100–159/109), repeat test for proteinuria by automated reader and if confirmed 1^+, requests protein-creatinine ratio (>30mg/mmol is significant)
- If > 30 mg/mmol, admit for surveillance
- Considers treatment with labetalol and states target blood pressure reading. NICE recommends treating moderate hypertension with labetalol, nifedipine or methyldopa
- Plan of care while in-patient (monitor BP four times a day; no need to repeat quantification of proteinuria etc.)
- Foetal scan for growth, amniotic fluid volume and umbilical artery Doppler.
- At 31 weeks of gestation, BP reading is 168/112 but Mrs Bergman remains asymptomatic. Foetal growth is satisfactory
- Severe hypertension (160/110 or higher) with or without pre-eclampsia requires critical care referral according to NICE guidelines, and requires definitive treatment
- Start anticonvulsant therapy, intravenous MgSO4. Not to use diazepam, phenytoin or lytic cocktail
- Start corticosteroids for foetal lung maturity. Dexamethasone or betamethasone
- Fluid balance chart. Limit maintenance fluids to 80ml/hour unless there are other ongoing fluid losses e.g. haemorrhage
- Inform Special Care Baby Unit
- Consider delivering the patient and discuss mode of delivery. Caesarean section vs Induction of labour (CS vs IOL)

Notes for Candidate

The scenario is taken from a common clinical scenario of our daily practice. It not only assesses the content of the knowledge given to the patient but also assesses your evidence-based knowledge.

Practice this scenario with one of your friends who can act as a role player of an assessor and ask another friend to provide you with feedback.

Further reading

Hypertension in pregnancy: diagnosis and management, Clinical guideline [CG107] Published date: August 2010 last updated: January 2011. https://www.nice.org.uk/guidance/cg107

Task 6 **Renal disease**

Instructions for Candidate

This task assesses the following clinical skills:

- Patient safety
- Communication with patients and their relatives
- Information gathering
- Applied clinical knowledge

You are an ST5 registrar in maternal medicine antenatal clinic and have been asked to see Helen Byrne for the first time. Helen is on anti- hypertensives secondary to a renal problem.

Take a history and plan her future pregnancy care.

You have 10 minutes for this task (+ 2mins initial reading time).

Instruction for Assessor

This task assesses the candidate's ability to take a focussed history and apply their knowledge in management of pregnancy in a woman with renal disease.

Please do not interrupt or prompt.

There are some marks on the process mark sheet for the actor to assign at the end of the station. Record your overall clinical impression of the candidate for each domain (i.e. should this performance be pass, borderline, or a fail).

Instructions for Role Player

You are Helen Byrne, aged 30. You are married to Frank and are both primary school teachers. This is your first pregnancy. You are 15 weeks pregnant. Your dating scan revealed a live singleton pregnancy and first trimester Down's syndrome screening gave a risk of 1:50,000.

You have had focal segment glomerulonephritis since you were 19. You have been managed with tablets to control your blood pressure with (Lisinopril 5mg) and this was changed to Methyldopa 500mg twice daily by your GP. Your recent blood pressure was 120/84. Your midwife has told you that you have protein in your urine. Your latest creatinine two weeks ago was 260iu/l. You are concerned about the effect of your kidney disease on your baby.

If specifically asked:

- You have never needed dialysis. Your kidney doctor has seen you at the beginning of pregnancy and has started you on Aspirin
- You are otherwise fit and well. No one else in your family has any kidney problems
- You have frequent water infections and have been on low dose oral antibiotics as a prophylaxis

Assessment

Marking Scheme		
Patient safety:		
Pass	Borderline	Fail
Communication with patients and their relatives:		
Pass	Borderline	Fail
Information gathering:		
Pass	Borderline	Fail
Applied clinical knowledge:		
Pass	Borderline	Fail

Notes for Marking

Patient safety

- Assesses the patient's main concerns and ideas
- Discusses the high risk nature of the pregnancy
- Discusses possible complications and measures to reduce them
- Involves patient in the process (e.g. encouraging them to express their ideas, or preferences)

Communication with patients and their relatives

- Greets, introduces self and role, checks patient's name
- Consent to proceed and explains nature of interview
- Assesses patient's starting point (what the patient wants to know) and sets the agenda
- Clear organized explanation in logical sequence
- Chunks: e.g. provides information in reasonable chunks
- Checks patient's understanding.
- Language (easily understood, avoids or explains jargon) although recognizes the patients knowledge of their condition
- Uses visual aids appropriately e.g. diagrams or uses analogies to aid explanation
- Presents a clear and succinct history to the assessor

Information gathering

- Obtains a relevant and focussed obstetric history
- Obtains patients views, ideas, expectations, and concerns regarding renal problem and anti hypertensives

Applied clinical Knowledge

- Demonstrates a sound and comprehensive evidence-based clinical knowledge
- Renal disease needs to be managed via a multidisciplinary approach involving renal physicians
- Women with a raised creatinine are at risk of pre-eclampsia and foetal growth restriction
- Serial four weekly growth scans from 24 weeks
- Alternate week assessment of BP and proteinuria.
- Creatinine levels to be done in each trimester
- Consider thromboprophylaxis antenatally if low serum albumin levels or significant proteinuria
- Preterm labour is common (both iatrogenic and spontaneous)
- Justify management plan

Notes for Candidate

Chronic renal disease can be classified according to creatinine levels with mild up to 125micromol/L, moderate 125–250micromol/L and severe >250micromol/L. Co-existing hypertension is common, with ACE inhibitors commonly used to control blood pressure (and reduce proteinuria).

Pre-pregnancy counselling is important to ensure that potential teratogenic drugs are converted to more 'pregnancy friendly' options. The outcome for the pregnancy is dependent on the BP control at booking, severity of hypertension, level of renal impairment and proteinuria along with the underlying cause of chronic renal disease.

Further reading

Pregnancy in women with renal disease, StratOG. https://stratog.rcog.org.uk/tutorial/renal-disease/pregnancy-in-women-with-renal-disease-6867

Task 7 **Autoimmune problems**

Instructions for Candidate

This task assesses the following clinical skills:

- Patient safety
- Communication with patients and their relatives
- Information gathering
- Applied clinical knowledge

You are about to see Naomi Jaden, 27 years old, who is known to have SLE for a few years. She is now married and the couple is planning to have a baby and is referred to you for pre-pregnancy counselling. Naomi was diagnosed with lupus nephritis three years ago after a renal biopsy. She is in good health for over 18 months and is quite keen on getting pregnant. However, she is very concerned about the effects of pregnancy on her disease because she has been through very rough times during her flares in the past. She is also keen to know how the disease may affect her baby at all.

This is a counselling station and the role-player will ask you several questions. You should address her concerns and provide a plan of management.

You have 10 minutes for this task (+ 2mins initial reading time).

Instructions for Assessor

This station assesses the candidate's communication skills and the application of knowledge regarding SLE in Pregnancy.

Please do not interrupt or prompt the candidates.

Record your overall clinical impression of the candidate for each domain (e.g. should this performance be pass, borderline, or a fail).

Instruction for Role Player

You are Naomi Jaden, 27 years old, and have never been pregnant before. You were diagnosed as SLE about six years ago when you were investigated for severe fatigue, aches in joints, skin rashes and cold fingers. The diagnosis was made by blood tests that tested positive for antibodies. A few years later your kidneys got affected by SLE. You have taken the treatment seriously after the diagnosis because you are very health conscious. You took the following medications in the past:

- Methotrexate
- Mycophenolate mofetil
- Rituximab
- Ramipril

for over 18 months now you have not had a flare and your medications have been changed. Presently you are taking the following medications:

- Hydroxycholoroquine
- Prednisolone
- Simvastatin
- Candesartan

You are also taking Iron and Vit D supplements regularly. You have recently have had a full range of tests done by your doctor and they have now referred you for advice on pregnancy because you are keen to have a family after getting married to David, your partner for ten years. You are aware that with your health condition pregnancy and delivery carries a higher risk but you welcome an opportunity to discuss your concerns with an obstetrician. You should ask the following questions to the candidate:

- What are the risks to my health if I get pregnant?
- How can my disease affect my baby?
- What measures can be taken to reduce the risks?
- What measures will be taken during pregnancy?
- Are my medications safe to be used during pregnancy?
- Can I have a home birth?

Temperament: You are a very careful person and like to develop a complete understanding of everything before embarking on a pregnancy. You are a composed but inquisitive person.

Ideas: You have some idea that the disease can flare up during pregnancy. You also have an idea that not all medications are safe during pregnancy and some of them might affect the development of baby.

Concerns: You have concerns regarding disease flare up because you have had quite hard time in the past coping with the symptoms. You used to be a healthcare worker but you stopped working ever since you developed this problem because you felt your performance at work is not 100%.

Expectations: You are expecting to have a clear understanding of your health condition and its implications on the pregnancy, so that you can make a decision on the right time to conceive. You also want to be prepared for the challenges pregnancy and motherhood might bring to you in reference to your disease.

Assessment

Marking Scheme

Patient safety:

Pass	Borderline	Fail

Communication with patients and their relatives:

Pass	Borderline	Fail

Information gathering:

Pass	Borderline	Fail

Applied clinical knowledge:

Pass	Borderline	Fail

Notes for Marking

Patient safety

- Demonstrates awareness of safety of investigations and therapeutics pre-conception, during pregnancy and in the postnatal including safe prescribing
- Demonstrates an understanding of both the impact of pregnancy on pre-existing conditions and the impact of those conditions on the foetus

Communicating with patients

- Ability to identify their concerns and expectations and be honest where there is clinical uncertainty
- Sharing information with the patient regarding the medical disorders and its impact on pregnancy and the foetus
- Be able to provide a clear plan of management and follow-up from pre pregnancy, early pregnancy, late pregnancy, delivery through the postpartum care
- Ability to emphasize the importance of multidisciplinary care

Information gathering

- Ability to take a concise and relevant medical history
- Skills in signposting and guiding the consultation
- Ensuring patient understanding and encouraging questions
- Ability to describe to the patient with co-existing medical disorders a clear action plan and the rationale for follow up based on the discussion

Applied clinical knowledge

- Knowledge of pre-conception, antenatal and postnatal care including the risks of maternal morbidity and mortality related to the medical co-morbidity

Notes for Candidate

This is a counselling station and you should aim to cover most of the following points:

- Assess disease activity and last remission
- Establish other organs involvement
- Check symptoms, BP, urine for protiens and blood, FBC (Full Blood Count), renal and liver functions)
- Check medications and assess if there are safer alternatives
- Arrange tests to assess the following: Echocardiogram if any symptoms suggestive of pulmonary hypertension or cardiomyopathy, lung function tests, Chest X-rays, Antibodies associated with adverse pregnancy outcomes (e.g. anti-Ro, anti-La, aPL, aCL, lupus anticoagulant, anti-β2 glycoprotein, anti-DNA and ANA)
- Offer routine pre pregnancy advice e.g. folic acid (increase to 5mg if patient is using antifolate medications, otherwise 400mcg/day)
- Identify risk factors that can be associated with adverse pregnancy outcome:
    - Active disease within six months prior to conception, during pregnancy or at first presentation during pregnancy
    - Active lupus nephritis (risk for foetal loss: 8–36%)
    - Other associated disorders: chronic hypertension, secondary antiphospholipid antibody syndrome, pre-existing renal disease and first trimester proteinuria levels of >500mg/day
    - Presence of antibodies:
        - secondary antiphospholipid antibody syndrome
        - double-stranded DNA antibodies.
        - presence of other antibodies (i.e. anti-Ro/anti-La; 2% risk of congenital heart block in the foetus)

- Biochemistry:
  - serum creatinine levels of >280mg/l at conception has a 70–80% risk of adverse pregnancy outcomes
  - thrombocytopenia
  - hypocomplementemia
- *Risks to mother:*
  - lupus flare
  - 20 fold increase risk of maternal death
  - Increased risk of pre-eclampsia and eclampsia
  - Increased risk of DVT, PE and stroke
  - Increased risk of C-section
- *Risks to foetus:*
  - Increased risk of miscarriage and still birth
  - Increased risk of preterm birth
  - Increased risk of IUGR
  - Neonatal death and neonatal Lupus.
- *Pre-pregnancy management*
  - Need to be booked under consultant and requires a multidisciplinary approach with input from consultant physician. Additional to routine pregnancy care, following should be added:
- *Antenatal care:*
  - Blood pressure—monthly monitoring, with a target blood pressure of <130/80mmHg)
  - Urine protein: creatinine ratio, full blood count, complement and renal function—be aware of possible nephritis flare, pre-eclampsia, haemolysis elevated liver enzymes and low platelets (HELLP) syndrome
  - Medication—administer aspirin 75mg, continue disease-modifying drugs if safe and consider need for thromboprophylaxis as clotting factors are reduced due to loss in proteinuria
- *Delivery:*
  - Mode of delivery—caesarean section is only indicated for obstetric reasons. If she is on steroids antenatally, need of intravenous steroids in labour
  - Time of delivery—there is an increased elective preterm delivery rate secondary to pre-eclampsia or foetal growth restriction
  - Postpartum—monitor blood pressure, renal function and follow-up
  - Foetal monitoring includes serial growth scans with umbilical artery doppler for foetal surveillance; uterine artery doppler is of no value

Further reading

Smyth, A., A Systematic Review and Meta-Analysis of Pregnancy Outcomes in Patients with Systemic Lupus Erythematosus and Lupus Nephritis, *Clinical Journal of the American Society of Nephrology* 5: 2060–8, 2010. doi:10.2215/CJN.00240110.

Task 8 **Haematological problems**

Instruction for Candidate

This task assesses the following clinical skills:

- Patient safety
- Communication with patients and their relatives
- Information gathering
- Applied clinical knowledge

You are an ST5 doctor working in the Antenatal Clinic and your next patient is Mrs. Louise James.

You are expected to take a history from the patient and make a plan of care for the remainder of her pregnancy. (See Box 10.1).

Box 10.1 Letter from GP

13th November 2015
Dear Obstetrician
RE: Mrs. Louise James DOB xx/xx/xxxx
Thank you for seeing Mrs. James for booking in her first pregnancy. Attached are her recent blood results.
Yours sincerely,
Dr Brown
GP

Date xx/xx/xxxx
Louise James
Date of Birth: dd/mm/yy
Hospital no: xyx

Thrombophilia Screen: 02.06.15
Protein C: 1.0 IU/ml (0.7–1.4IU/ml)
Protein S: 0.2 IU/ml (0.7–1.25IU/ml)
Factor V Leiden: Normal
Antithrombin: 1.1 IU/ml (0.8–1.2IU//ml)

Date xx/xx/xxxx
Louise James
Date of Birth: dd/mm/yy
Hospital no: xyx

Thrombophilia Screen: 14.04.15
Protein C: 0.9 IU/ml (0.7–1.4IU/ml)
Protein S: 0.3 IU/ml (0.7–1.25IU/ml)
Factor V Leiden: Normal
Antithrombin: 1.1 IU/ml (0.8–1.2IU/ml)

You have 10 minutes for this task (+ 2mins initial reading time).

Instruction for Assessor

Allow the candidate to conduct the consultation uninterrupted. The patient has been referred to ANC for booking.

Instruction for Role Player

You are Louise James, aged 32. You work as an investment banker in London and are married to Lewis. This is your third pregnancy; you had a termination when you were 23 and your second pregnancy ended in a miscarriage two years ago, you have been trying to conceive since then. You had just had your first private consultation regarding IVF when you discovered a week later that you were pregnant again.

Concerns: You are worried that you will have another miscarriage. Although you are expecting that the doctor will recommend heparin injections you are worried about the effect that these will have on your baby; your sister's baby was born prematurely at 33 weeks and you are worried that it may have been due to the treatment she was given.

Expectations: You expect the doctor to recommend treatment with heparin.

You expect the doctor to explain the risks and benefits of the treatment in particular the harm it would cause to the baby and the risks of premature labour. Following your previous miscarriage you saw a gynaecologist privately to request further investigations; this was when it was discovered that you have a thrombophilia.

If you are specifically asked:

- Your last menstrual period was 11 September
- You had a private ultrasound last week which gives your EDD as 17 June 2016 and confirmed that the baby was fine
- Your periods are regular and your smears are up to date
- You have had two previous pregnancies, one surgical termination when you were 23 years old and a miscarriage two years ago. The miscarriage was found when you had bleeding and a scan showed no heartbeat at six weeks; you had treatment with tablets
- You have no medical problems and apart from the termination you have never had any operations. You have never had a deep vein thrombosis or pulmonary embolism
- You do not take any regular medication but have been taking pregnancy multivitamins for the last two years. You are not allergic to any medications
- Your sister had a blood clot, a DVT, in her first pregnancy; you don't know whether she has been tested for clotting disorders. No one else in your family has had blood clots
- You do not smoke, and you stopped drinking alcohol as soon as you had a positive pregnancy test, you previously drank six units a week

Temperament: You are anxious but this is expressed as being abrupt with the doctor. You are used to being in control and are worried about not knowing what will happen in this pregnancy. If the doctor approaches you in a respectful way and diffuses your anxieties, you become calmer for the rest of the consultation.

Ideas: You are expecting that the doctor will recommend treatment with heparin injections as your sister had this in her second pregnancy.

You are expecting to have an epidural in your labour and are concerned when the doctor tells you that this may not be possible, if the doctor does not spontaneously mention a plan for labour you can ask if you are able to have an epidural

Assessment

Marking Scheme

Patient safety:

Pass	Borderline	Fail

Communication with patients and their relatives:

Pass	Borderline	Fail

Information gathering:

Pass	Borderline	Fail

Applied clinical knowledge:

Pass	Borderline	Fail

Notes for Marking

Patient safety

- Elicits patient's main concerns and ideas: risk of blood clot, worries about premature labour with heparin, concerns about labour analgesia
- Gives explanation of recommended treatment and address concerns
- Negotiates a mutually agreed, acceptable, safe plan
- Acknowledges anxieties and diffuses situation

Communication with patients and their relatives

- Greets, introduced self and role, checks patient identity
- Consent to proceed and explains nature of consultation
- Assesses patient's starting point and sets agenda
- Clear, organized history in a logical sequence
- Chunks: provides information in reasonable chunks specific to patient's level of understanding
- Checks patient's understanding
- Language: easily understood, avoids or explains jargon
- Communicates clear plan for future care and ensures patient understands

Information gathering

Obtains a relevant and focussed obstetrics and medical history.

Obtains patients views, ideas, expectations, and concerns regarding her situation.

Applied clinical knowledge

The history should cover the following:

Pregnancy:

LMP

Any ultrasound thus far

O and G history: one surgical termination of pregnancy, one miscarriage, history of subfertility, smears normal

PMH: none, no personal history of VTE

PSH: surgical termination of pregnancy

Medications: none

Family history: sister: oestrogen provoked DVT, no other family members with a history of VTE

SH: non-smoker, stopped alcohol

Demonstrates a sound and comprehensive evidence based knowledge.

Demonstrates clear understanding of thromboprophylaxis in pregnancy.

Performs VTE risk assessment:

High risk thrombophilia (Protein S deficiency)—Score 3

First degree relative with oestrogen provoked VTE—Score 1

Total score—4

With a total score of ≥ 4 antenatal thromboprophylaxis should be considered from the first trimester with LMWH according to weight.

The treatment should commence as soon as practicably possible; ideally the candidate should provide the patient with a prescription within the consultation. Make provisions for the patient to be taught how to administer treatment and dispose of sharps.

Refer to nominated trust expert.

Talks about labour implications: advise that if any bleeding or signs of labour should prompt cessation of LMWH.

Regional anaesthesia should be avoided for at least 12 hours following the previous dose of LMWH.

Offer referral to anaesthetic team for antenatal review.

The patient should have 6 weeks of postnatal thromboprophylaxis; safe with breastfeeding.

Justifies management recommended.

Notes for Candidate

This scenario is testing your ability to take a thorough history and apply the knowledge in order to plan the care for the antenatal period, labour and postnatal period.

Further reading

Thrombosis and Embolism during Pregnancy and the Puerperium, Reducing the Risk (Green-top Guideline No. 37a). https://www.rcog.org.uk/en/guidelines-research-services/guidelines/gtg37a/

Task 9 **Vulnerable women**

Instructions for Candidate

This task assesses the following clinical skills:

- Patient safety
- Communication with patients and their relatives
- Information gathering
- Applied clinical knowledge

You are a ST5 doctor working in the delivery suite triage and are asked to see Wendy Haines, a 36-year-old woman who is 30 weeks pregnant and presenting with non-specific abdominal pain. She has attended with her three children. The midwife in charge informs you that she is worried about this woman as it is her fifth admission to triage with the same complaint over the last four weeks. Please take a full history and when you are ready, ask the assessor for the examination findings and the results of the investigations that were taken. After you have been given this information, you will be able to ask Wendy some further questions about the findings. You will be asked to discuss the diagnosis of her problem and suggest a management plan.

You have 10 minutes for this task (+ 2mins initial reading time).

Instructions for Assessor

Please read the instructions to the candidate and actor.

After the candidate has finished taking the history, they will ask you for the examination findings and results of investigations.

Examination findings:

Soft, non-tender, abdomen with a gravid uterus, SFH = 29cms that plots on the twentieth centile of her customized GROW chart.

A large bruise noted is in the left upper quadrant below the breast (appears yellowish in colour) and a smaller, blue bruise in the suprapubic region. There are three discreet lesions on the left side of the neck that are about 5–10mm in diameter that appear to be forming a scab.

Speculum NAD

Investigations:

FBC, U and Es, LFTs and CRP within normal limits

Urine analysis NAD

CTG normal for 30/40

Once all this information has been given to the candidate, they should ask Wendy how the bruising and lesions were sustained.

Instructions for Role Player

You are Wendy Haines, aged 32, married to Richard who is a submariner in the Navy and away at sea for long intervals. He is currently on shore leave and has been at home for the last six weeks. Your relationship is not good and you always hate it when he is home on leave and try to avoid being in his company. You have three children together; Daisy aged six, David aged four and Duncan 18 months—all normal vaginal deliveries, but Daisy was born at 34 weeks, small for gestational age and had to spend three weeks in the neonatal unit for respiratory problems. They are all fit and well, but David has to see a psychologist for treatment of his ADHD. You are concerned as you have been having some moderate abdominal pain for the last few weeks. You feel it in the left upper side of your bump and aware of slight increased urinary frequency. There has been no vaginal discharge, bowels are moving well and there have been good foetal movements. Other than well controlled asthma you are otherwise healthy. You do not take any medication, but took citalopram for postpartum depression after the birth of David. You were medicated for a year before your mood improved and you decided to stop taking the medication. You are not allergic to any medication, you have no family history; you do not smoke nor drink alcohol. You struggle financially as you rely on your husband's income alone as you are a full time mother. You have been seen four times over the last few weeks and you do not feel that the doctors who have assessed you before have really identified the cause of your problems.

After the candidate has been given information about your injuries, they should ask you how the injuries were sustained. At this point you disclose that you frequently have fights that result in Richard punching you in the face and abdomen. He has forced you to have sex in the past when you did not want to have it. When he gets really mad, he burns you with his cigarettes.

Temperament: Your manner is very important during this role play. Avoid eye contact with the candidate and look subdued. Keep pulling your collar up around your neck as you are trying to hide cigarette burns that are on your left side of your neck.

Ideas: You hope that this doctor will finally notice that you are distressed as don't know what help to ask for or how to get yourself out of the violent relationship.

Concerns: You are concerned that Richard will kill you if he finds out that you have told someone about his physically violent attacks towards you.

Assessment

Marking Scheme

Patient safety:

Pass	Borderline	Fail

Communication with patients and their relatives:

Pass	Borderline	Fail

Information gathering:

Pass	Borderline	Fail

Applied clinical knowledge:

Pass	Borderline	Fail

Notes for Marking

Patient safety

- Assesses the patient's main concerns and ideas
- Aware of red flag disclosure of physical violence—this has to have an action plan (contact one of more of the following; consultant on-call/ adult safeguarding team/ local domestic violence services for advice)
- Patient and her children must not leave the hospital until a plan for safety made
- Is open and honest with patient

- Explain that confidentiality might have to be breached on a 'need to know' basis to trigger safeguarding cascade

Communication with patients and their relatives

- Greets, introduces self and role, checks patient's name
- Consent to undertake consultation
- Consultation performed in a sensitive manner
- Language (easily understood, avoids or explains jargon)
- Presents a clear and succinct history to the assessor

Information gathering

- Obtains a relevant and focussed obstetric history
- Obtains patients views, ideas, expectations, and concerns
- History of mental health problems
- Children: history of behavioural problems
- Obtains history in a sensitive manner

Applied clinical knowledge

- Unexplained bruises, especially those a differing stages of healing
- Injuries to areas covered by clothing (on abdomen)
- Repeat visits to maternity services
- Presentation with a vague complaint
- History of SFGA (could also include miscarriage and/or IUD)
- Identifies that the diagnosis is domestic violence
- Aware of the signs of domestic violence
- Aware that this is a high risk pregnancy an she will need surveillance in a consultant led antenatal clinic

Notes for Candidate

Domestic violence is often a difficult subject for the patient to broach with health care professionals. Once it is disclosed it is a red flag and has to be acted upon. You might not know what to do, but doing nothing is not an option. There is always an on-call consultant, domestic violence helplines, safeguarding teams or even the police to ask for help.

Once it is disclosed, the pregnancy becomes high risk as there is an increase of miscarriage, small for gestational age foetus and IUD in this cohort of patients. The patient will need surveillance in a consultant led antenatal clinic because of the increased risk of poor obstetric outcomes.

Further reading

NICE guideline 50. Domestic Violence and Abuse: Multiagency working February 2014. https://www.womensaid.org.uk/

Mezey GC., Bewley S, Domestic Violence and Pregnancy. *BMJ* 1997; 314: 1295.

Task 10 **Psychiatric problems**

Instructions for Candidate

This task assesses the following clinical skills:

- Patient safety
- Communication with patients and their relatives
- Information gathering
- Applied clinical knowledge

You are a ST4 doctor working in the antenatal clinic. You are about to have a booking visit consultation with Sadie Upton, a 26-year-old primigravida who has been referred for consultant led care with her medical history of depression. She has maintained a good and stable mood for the past five years by taking 40mg fluoxetine once daily. She had a brief trial without antidepressants ten months ago, but this led to a relapse of severe depression that required admission to a psychiatric hospital for one month.

Sadie wishes to know more about the safety of her medication in pregnancy. She is particularly keen to know of any significant risks to her unborn child as she would consider discontinuing the medication if it could cause the child harm.

You have 10 minutes for this task (+ 2mins initial reading time).

Instructions for Assessor

Please read the instructions to the candidate and the actor.

This OCE assesses the candidate's communication skills and application of knowledge regarding psychotropic medications in pregnancy.

Please do not interrupt or prompt.

Record your overall clinical impression of the candidate for each domain (e.g. should this performance be pass, borderline, or a fail).

Instructions for Role Player

You are Sadie Upton and have just had your dating scan and you are very happy to discover you are 13 weeks pregnant. You have suffered with severe depression for the last seven years. Initially your GP referred you for counselling with a psychologist, however you felt this intervention made your symptoms worse. You have tried a few classes of antidepressant, but have enjoyed good mental health using SSRIs, especially fluoxetine for the past five years. When you stop taking the medication you get very severe depression that has resulted in admission under the Mental Health Act to a psychiatric hospital for electroconvulsive therapy (ECT). You are otherwise fit and well with no other medical problems. You do not smoke, nor take recreational drugs and you consume about one to two units of alcohol each week. You work as a hairdresser and you have been in a stable relationship with your partner Martin Fraser for the past two years. You are both delighted at the prospect of becoming parents.

Temperament: You are very excited about the pregnancy, but have become worried you might be damaging your unborn baby with the strong medication you take. You are not a risk taker and would not gamble with something as important as your child's health.

Ideas: You think you will be told that your fears are correct and you should stop taking the medication straightaway.

Concerns: You are worried about what will happen to your mental health if you stop the medication. However, you are more concerned about any harm the medication might cause to your unborn child.

Expectations: You want the doctor to explain:

- The benefit of continuing the medication throughout pregnancy
- Are there any harmful effects of the medication to the unborn baby?
- Will the medication have any long term effects on the child?
- Will any additional maternal or foetal monitoring be required?
- Is it safe to breast feed using fluoxetine?

If the doctor explains it is safe and important to continue the medication, engage well with the consultation by asking these questions.

If the doctor suggests you stop the medication as it is dangerous to the baby, start to cry inconsolably and explain you couldn't bear the thought of going back to the psychiatric hospital. Only allow the consultation to continue if the doctor retracts the statement and says it is safe to take and continues the consultation.

At the end, you will award some marks according to how well the candidate addressed your questions and concerns.

Assessment

Marking Scheme

Patient safety:

Pass Borderline Fail

Communication with patients and their relatives:

Pass Borderline Fail

Information gathering:

Pass Borderline Fail

Applied clinical knowledge:

Pass Borderline Fail

Notes for Marking

Patient safety

- Elicits patient's ideas and concerns
- Given the patient's past admission for treatment under the Mental Health Act ensures that she knows the importance of continuing the medication and only stopping it under the advice and monitoring by a psychiatrist

Communication with patients and their relatives

- Greets, introduces self and role, checks patient's name
- Consent to proceed and explains nature of the consultation
- Assesses patient's starting point (attending clinic to discuss medication) and sets the agenda
- Clear organized explanation in logical sequence
- Chunks: i.e. provides information in reasonable chunks

- Checks patient's understanding of the benefits and risk of the medication
- Language (easily understood, avoids or explains jargon)

Information gathering

- Obtains a relevant and focussed obstetric history
- Obtains patients views, ideas, expectations, and concerns
- History of mental health problems
- Obtains history in a sensitive manner

Applied clinical knowledge

- Demonstrates evidence based clinical knowledge of safety of SSRIs in pregnancy
- Common class of mediation taken during pregnancy
- The risk to the mother of unstable mental health far outweigh the benefit to the foetus of stopping fluoxetine i.e. deterioration of mental health that could lead to:

Maternal

  - Self-neglect
  - Relationship problems (partner, other children, wider family and friends)
  - Poor engagement with employment
  - Increased hospital admission with non-specific obstetric problems
  - Suicide—still common cause of indirect maternal death
- ***Foetal***
  - Increased risk of preterm delivery, SFGA (thought to be related to long term maternal cortisol release from sustained psychological stress and IUD)
  - Neglect and harm once born
  - Failure to meet milestones
  - Increased risk of problem behaviour, hyperactivity, inattention and peer problems
  - Other than slight increased risk of postpartum haemorrhage, to additional risk of use of SSRIs to mother in pregnancy
  - Extensive research has failed to show any significant detrimental effect in utero —slight increased risk of persistent pulmonary hypertension of the newborn (PPHN)
  - No robust evidence that it leads to neonatal abstinence syndrome (NAS)
  - There is some concern that the use of paroxetine is associated with cardiac malformations, but meta analyses have not demonstrated an statistically significant increase in the risk of malformation
  - Big studies show there is no long term effects on fetus of SSRI use in pregnancy (motor or behavioural skills)
  - No additional foetal monitoring needed unless other risk factors to indicate serial ultrasound scans
  - Maternal mood need to be monitored by asking the Whooley questions (see appendix) at each and every antenatal contact with midwives, GPs and obstetricians. If the woman responds yes to any two of the three questions then a referral need to make for a formal psychiatric assessment
  - Fluoxetine is safe to use during breast feeding. Some is excreted into breast milk, but it is not thought to be expressed in a significant quantity to have any effect or be harmful to the baby.
  - Counsels the patient with relevant information that is factually correct
  - Makes a mutually acceptable plan to continue fluoxetine throughout pregnancy and the postpartum period, even if breastfeeding

Notes for Candidate

This consultation is extremely common in perinatal mental health antenatal clinics. The format of this task is to assess both communication knowledge of safety of SSRIs in pregnancy. It is vital to give the patient accurate and concise information; your delivery should be in a sensitive manner.

Undertaking this communication task can be particularly stressful as you get *subjective marks* from the role players. Therefore, to overcome the additional nerves associated with these stations practice, practice speaking aloud giving explanations, even if it is just to your living room wall! Get other colleagues to help you with this station to provide you with feedback and how they would have scored you on those all-important subjective marks.

Further reading

Antenatal and postnatal mental health: clinical management and service guidance. NICE clinical guideline 192. December 2014.

Grzeskowiak LE, Morrison JL, Henriksen TB, Bech BH, Obel C, Olsen J, Pedersen LH. Prenatal antidepressant exposure and child behavioural outcomes at 7 years of age: a study within the Danish National Birth Cohort. *BJOG: An International Journal of Obstetrics & Gynaecology* 2015; DOI: 10.1111/1471-0528.13611.

Grzeskowiak LE, McBain R, Dekker GA, Cliftona VL. Antidepressant use in late gestation and risk of postpartum haemorrhage: a retrospective cohort study. *BJOG: An International Journal of Obstetrics & Gynaecology,* 2015; DOI 10.1111.1471-0528.13612.

Handal M, Skurtveit S, Furu K, Hernandez-Diaz S, Skovlund E, Nystad W, Selmer R. Motor development in children prenatally exposed to selective serotonin reuptake inhibitors: a large population-based pregnancy cohort study. *BJOG: An International Journal of Obstetrics & Gynaecology*, 2015; DOI: 10.1111/1471-0528.13582.

Wilson KL, Zelig CM, Harvey JP, Cunningham BS, Dolinsky BM, Napolitano PG. Persistent pulmonary hypertension of the newborn is associated with mode of delivery and not with maternal use of selective serotonin reuptake inhibitors. *American Journal of Perinatology*, 2011; 28: 19–24.

Chapter 11 **Management of labour**

Task 1 **Management of labour**

Instructions for Candidate

This task assesses the following clinical skills:

- Patient safety
- Communication with patients and their relatives
- Information gathering
- Applied clinical knowledge

You are a ST5 doctor in the antenatal clinic. You are asked to see Lucy Rogers who is a 32-year-old lady in her second pregnancy. She is currently 21 weeks pregnant with a normal detailed ultrasound scan of her baby. She is booked under consultant care having had shoulder dystocia (SD) with her first child Molly two years ago. You have had a chance to review the previous delivery records. Mrs Rogers had an uneventful pregnancy and normal labour. The baby's head delivered normally but then had a shoulder dystocia which required McRoberts manoeuvre and suprapubic pressure for delivery of the anterior shoulder. Molly weighed 3.5 kilogrammes with Apgar scores of seven and ten at one and ten minutes. The head to body delivery interval was three minutes. She is developing normally with appropriate milestones.

Mrs Rogers is very apprehensive about having another shoulder dystocia as it was very traumatic experience. She is seeking reassurance but also quite disappointed that this was not predicted and a proper explanation was not provided at the time.

You have 10 minutes for this task (+ 2mins initial reading time).

Instruction for Assessors

Please read instruction to candidate and role player

After initial consultation about the previous pregnancy and SD, tell the candidate that Mrs Rogers is keen to avoid a caesarean section and wants to go ahead with a vaginal delivery.

Ask the candidate to explain the options of mode of delivery to Mrs Rogers along with pros and cons. What can be done to prevent this and what is the course of action if it happens again? Can you provide reassurance?

Instructions for Role Player

You are Lucy Rogers, 32-year-old mother of two-year-old Molly. You had a straightforward pregnancy with Molly and a normal delivery which was unfortunately complicated by shoulder dystocia (difficulty in delivery of the baby's shoulders after delivery of the head). Although, Molly is doing absolutely fine and growing normally, you are extremely worried about having another shoulder dystocia (SD). It was all very traumatic experience for you and your husband Nick. You are also disappointed and slightly annoyed that this was not predicted and no proper explanation was provided at that time.

You are currently 21 weeks pregnant and just had the detailed scan of your baby. You are delighted that everything is normal. You have been sent round to the antenatal clinic to discuss your reasons for anxiety and plan for delivery in this pregnancy.

Temperament: You think you are mostly a calm, level headed sensible woman, but you like to be organized, well informed with a definite plan.

Ideas: You want an apology and an explanation as to why you were not warned about the possibility of SD with Molly and no proper explanation were offered after the event.

You are not keen for a caesarean section (CS) but want some reassurance with regards to proceeding with normal vaginal delivery.

Concerns: You want what is best for the baby but keen to avoid CS. You are apprehensive of being in similar emergency situation with the baby's shoulders getting stuck. Nick found it very traumatic as well.

Expectations: You want the doctor to explain:

- What is SD?
- Why SD happened last time?
- Why it was not predicted?
- Why you were not warned?
- When can you have a SD?
- Why it was not explained properly afterwards?

You want for a normal delivery but want to know:

- What are the chances of it happening again?
- What are the risks to the baby?
- Can something be done to reduce the chances of it happening again?
- What are your options regarding delivery?
- Would inducing labour early prevent SD?
- How will it be managed if it happens again?
- Can a CS be done once it is diagnosed?

Assessment

Marking scheme

Patient safety:

Pass Borderline Fail

Communication with patients and their relatives:

Pass Borderline Fail

Information gathering:

Pass Borderline Fail

Applied clinical knowledge:

Pass Borderline Fail

Notes for Marking

Patient safety

- Assesses patient's main concerns and ideas
- Gives options and discusses the pros and cons of each

- Involves patient in the process (encourages them to express their ideas or preferences)
- Negotiates a mutually agreed, acceptable and safe management plan, to be finalised nearer to term
- Open and honest
- Offer an apology
- Explain fully what has happened before and the chances of it happening again along with the possible complications
- Ensures that proper protocol will be followed if it happens along with filling an incident form and investigating the management.

Communication with patients and their relatives

- Greets, introduces self and role, checks patient's name
- Consent to proceed and explains nature of the interview
- Assesses what patient wants to know (starting point) and sets the agenda
- Clear organised explanation in logical sequence
- Chunks: i.e. provides information in reasonable chunks
- Checks patients understanding
- Language (easily understood, avoids or explains jargon)
- Uses visual aids (e.g. diagrams) and analogies to aid explanation

Information gathering

- Obtains a relevant obstetric history
- Obtains the vital information from the notes
- Obtains the patients views, expectations, and concerns

Applied clinical knowledge

- Demonstrates a sound and comprehensive evidence based comprehensive knowledge
- Counsels the patient with relevant information that is factually correct
- Makes a robust and safe management plan taking patient's views into account

Notes for Candidate

Explanation of SD

- SD means that the baby requires additional manoeuvres for the delivery of the shoulders after the head has delivered and gentle traction has failed to deliver the rest of the body
- Can happen in 0.50–0.70% of deliveries
- Risk factors—diabetes, big baby, prolonged labour, epidural analgesia, previous shoulder dystocia
- Can be associated with significant complications of the mother and the baby
- Complications in mother can be significant bleeding after delivery 11% (postpartum haemorrhage), tear involving the muscles around the anal opening 3.8% (third and fourth degree tear)
- Most important complication of the baby is brachial plexus injury 2.3–16% of deliveries. Most of them resolve without permanent disability. Less than 10% result in permanent neurological disability

Previous delivery

- Apologies

- Difficult to predict SD especially in a straight forward pregnancy. Risk assessments are insufficiently predictive to allow prevention in majority of the cases
- Can happen without any risk factors
- There was no reason to suspect SD in a normal pregnancy with normal size baby
- No signs indicative of SD was picked up during labour or after delivery of the head
- Signs of diagnosing SD

Options

- Options are vaginal birth or elective caesarean section (CS)– either can be appropriate
- Second deliveries are usually easier than the first one but
- Difficult to predict recurrence of SD
- Previous SD is a risk factor—recurrence rate between 1–25%
- CS is a major surgery with known complications, some common complications and some rare but serious complications
- Induction of labour does not prevent SD in a non-diabetic woman even with suspected big baby
- Plan to be finalised nearer to term taking estimated foetal weight into account

Delivery

- All birth attendants will be aware of the methods for diagnosing SD and the techniques required to facilitate delivery
- Birth attendants will be vigilant for signs of SD
- If it is diagnosed, it will be managed in a structured way
- Immediately after recognition help will be called. So expect to see quite a few people in the room
- May need to make a cut for the manoeuvres if not had it already
- May need internal manoeuvres
- May have to go on all fours position
- Once baby delivered, will be handed over to the paediatricians immediately
- Extremely rarely need to break baby's clavicle bone, push the head in and do a caesarean section or divide the ligaments over symphysis pubis bone to deliver baby

Further reading

Green-top Guideline No. 42 2nd edition | March 2012 Shoulder Dystocia, RCOG. https://www.rcog.org.uk/globalassets/documents/guidelines/gtg_42.pdf

Task 2 **Intrapartum CTG**

Instructions for Candidate

This task assesses the following clinical skills:

- Patient safety
- Communication with colleagues
- Information gathering
- Applied clinical knowledge

You are the ST-4 doctor working as a registrar on-call for the delivery suite. In Room 5 Mrs Julie Smith has just been transferred from the midwifery-led unit for failure to progress. Mrs Julie Smith is 28 years old, in her first pregnancy with an uneventful antenatal period. There is no significant medical or surgical history of note. At 41 weeks and two days she is admitted with spontaneously ruptured membranes at 4cm cervical dilatation. Four hours later she is 5cm of cervical dilation.

Fig 11.1 is the CTG that is given to you. Please interpret the CTG, outline your management plan and describe to the assessor the actions to be taken. Should you need any other information please ask the assessor.

Next you are presented with a second CTG (Fig 11.2) taken four hours later. Please interpret the CTG and describe the actions to be taken.

Next you are asked to review the CTG taken four hours later (Fig 11.3), after one hour of pushing. Please interpret the CTG and describe the actions to be taken.

You have 10 minutes for this task (+ 2mins initial reading time). Allocate around 3 minutes for each of the 3 CTGs.

This station does not have a role player.

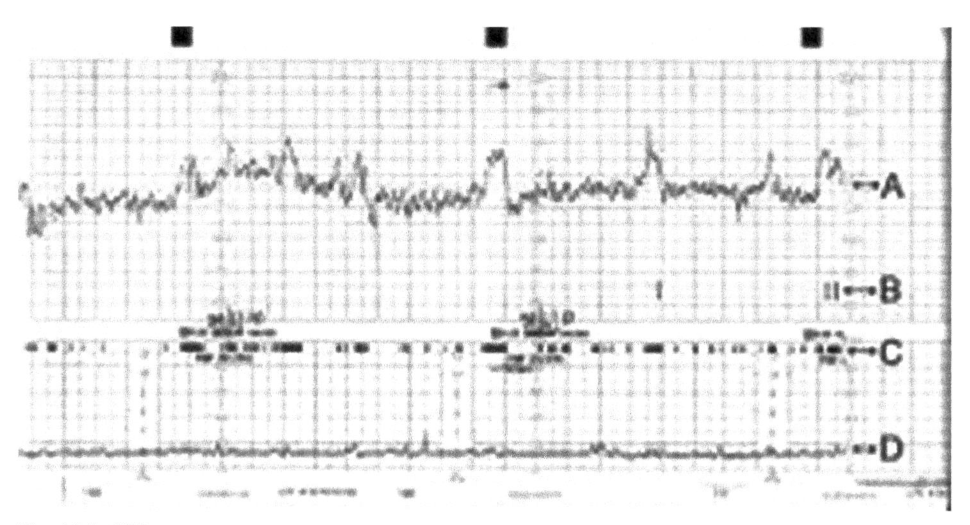

Fig. 11.1 CTG

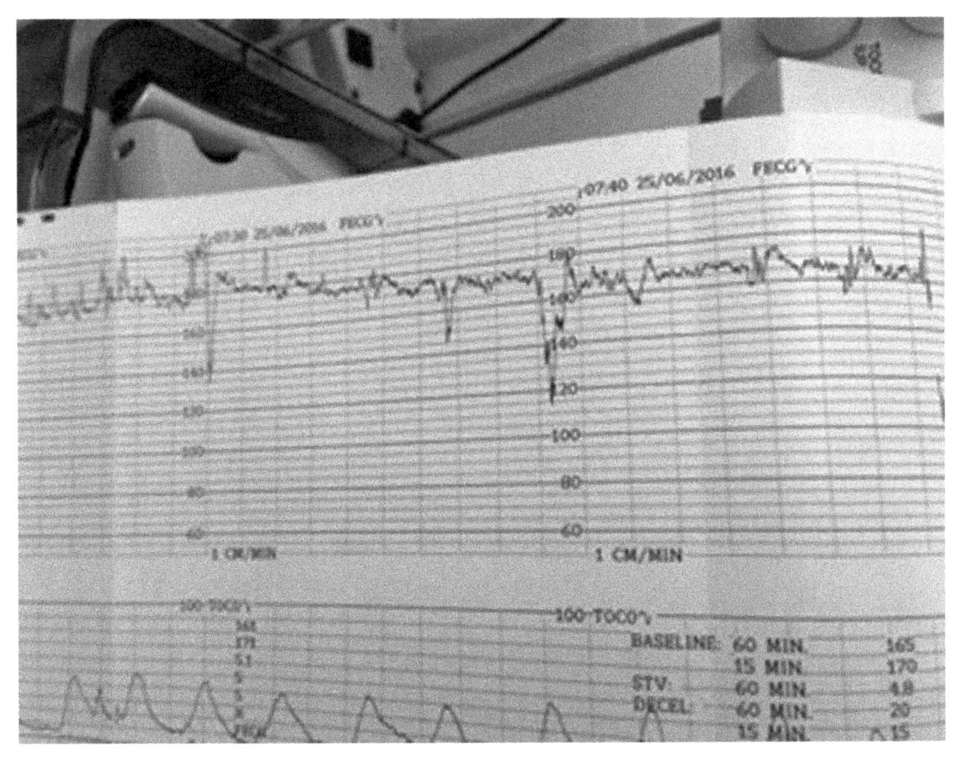

Fig. 11.2 CTG

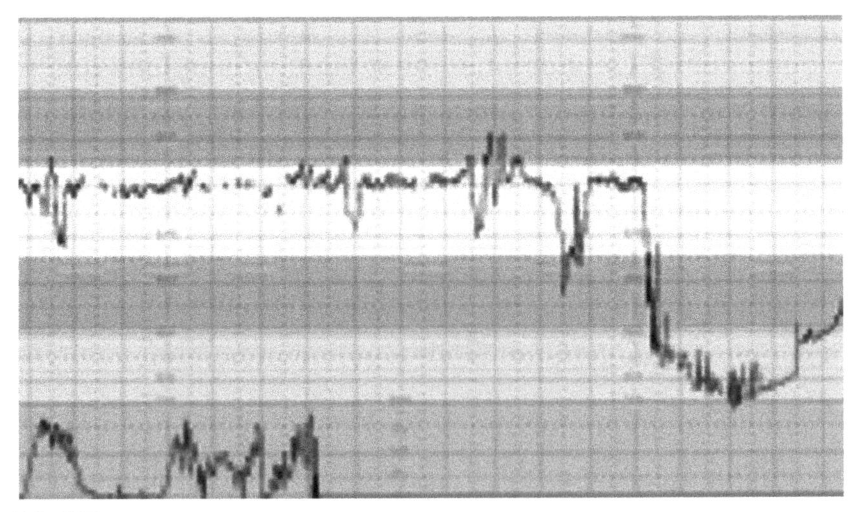

Fig. 11.3 CTG

Instructions for Assessor

Record your clinical impression (Pass, Borderline, or Fail) for the candidate on each of the domains.

Assessment

Marking Scheme

Patient safety:

Pass	Borderline	Fail

Communication with colleagues:

Pass	Borderline	Fail

Information gathering:

Pass	Borderline	Fail

Applied clinical knowledge:

Pass	Borderline	Fail

Notes for Marking

Patient safety

- Depending on the situation, able to interpret the CTG and put safe measures in place
- Does not guess and may ask for help if unable to interpret or make a decision

Communication with colleagues

- Clear and concise description of the CTG-s and the management plan

Information gathering

- Obtains relevant information required to contextualize the CTG prior to interpretation
- Able to interpret the CTG-s

Applied clinical knowledge

Part 1—Normal CTG

- The candidate diagnoses the delay in the first stage of labour according to the NICE criteria
- Offers support, hydration and effective pain relief
- Proposes Syntocinon for labour augmentation
- Explains that Oxytocin will bring forward the time of birth, but will not influence the mode of birth
- States regimen of oxytocin—the time between increments of the dose is no more frequent than every 30 minutes. Increase oxytocin until there are four to five contractions in ten minutes
- Explains the need for continuous CTG monitoring with the Syntocinon
- Offers the explanation of epidural analgesia as the Syntocinon has been given to bring about stronger uterine contractions and thereby more painful contractions
- Interprets the CTG as normal by taking a systematic approach—DR C BRAVADO
- Categorises each feature of CTG into normal, non-reassuring or abnormal

- Comments on the uterine activity
- Correctly interprets the CTG as normal

Part 2—Suspicious or non-reassuring CTG

- Comments on the CTG as suspicious by taking a systematic approach
- Categorizes each feature into normal, non-reassuring or abnormal
- Comments on uterine activity
- Correctly interprets the CTG as **suspicious** or in need of conservative measures.
- Requests information on cervical dilatation and fetal descent
- Is able to elucidate the causes of uncomplicated fetal tachycardia
- Suggests conservative measures of:
  - Checking temperature and maternal pulse
  - Offering paracetamol
  - Left lateral position
  - Oral or intravenous fluids
- Allow for variation in management of Syntocinon (either continuing or discontinuing is acceptable) as there are accelerations, which decreases the risk of foetal acidosis

Part 3—Pathological CTG or Abnormal CTG needing urgent intervention

- Interprets the CTG as pathological by taking a systematic approach—DR C BRAVADO
- Categorises each feature of the CTG into normal, non-reassuring or abnormal
- Comments on uterine activity, correctly interprets the CTG as pathological or needing urgent intervention
- Suggests ventouse delivery: allow for outlet forceps delivery.
- Ensure that the candidate is aware that the FBS is not appropriate for bradycardia
- Understands that conditions (LOA, + 2, no moulding) are favourable for instrumental vaginal delivery in the room.

Notes for Candidate

This is a CTG interpreting station. Please adopt a systematic approach.

DR C BRAVADO is the one that is commonly used however as long as you cover all the features you would be awarded the marks. DR is for determine risk. C is for contraction. BR is for baseline rate. A is for accelerations. VA is for variability. D is for decelerations. O is for the overall impression.

Go through each feature categorising it as: normal, non-reassuring or abnormal.

Comment on the uterine activity.

Give your overall impression. Comment on the association, where possible, with foetal physiology.

Following either NICE guidelines of either 2007 or 2014 is acceptable. Justification of your decision is what matters.

Distribute your time evenly between the 3 CTGS. Do not spend too much time on any one CTG. You will have to pass all 3 CTGs for a pass in the entire station. A failure in any one CTG will equate to failing the whole station.

Further reading

CTG interpretation and further management, StratOG. https://stratog.rcog.org.uk/tutorial/obstetrics/ctg-interpretation-and-further-management-6354

Task 3 **Intrauterine transfer**

Instructions for Candidate

This task assesses the following clinical skills:

- Patient safety
- Communication with patients and their relatives
- Information gathering
- Applied clinical knowledge

You are a ST5 doctor working on a twilight shift on delivery suite in a busy district general hospital with level 2 neonatal unit facilities. Your colleague has handed over to you at 5.00 pm. Mrs Patricia Mason is in her second pregnancy at 30 weeks with twins presenting with irregular tightening since 11.00 am that morning. One of the twins is known to have double bubble on scan at 20 weeks. The plan had been for delivery in a tertiary unit with paediatric surgical facilities. Your colleague has had a busy shift and has been unable to review her. She has been admitted since an hour. You have been asked to review her by the consultant on call with a view to arranging in utero transfer. Her husband and mother are unhappy that she has not been seen since admission

You have 10 minutes for this task (+ 2mins initial reading time).

Instructions for Role Player

You are Patricia, a 36-year-old mother of six-year-old Olivia who is fit and well. You had a straight forward pregnancy and delivered by caesarean section as the labour did not progress well and baby was lying back to back. You have a vague recollection of having got to 8cm in labour and needing a drip for contractions. You have had a miscarriage at eight weeks four years ago.

You are currently 30 weeks pregnant in your second ongoing pregnancy with twins. You have been told they have separate placentae. One of the twins has been diagnosed with problems with their stomach and you have been told that the there may be a blockage to the stomach and baby will need to be delivered in a specialist unit for surgery after delivery. No concerns were raised about the second twin. You are expecting a girl and a boy. You declined the needle test to check for Downs's syndrome as you have a low risk result from the screening programme. On your previous scans the doctors have informed you that there is more water around the boy and he has a possible blockage of his gut pipe around between the stomach and the small bowels.

The doctor assesses you and should explain that you at risk of going into preterm labour. Following an examination, the doctor confirms that your waters have not gone but they do a special test to check if you are in labour. You should be offered a scan to check how both the babies are lying. This is important to decide the mode of delivery.

The doctor should explain the plan of care for you and the babies. You will need to be transferred to another unit. Your booking hospital does not have the facilities to look after babies born before 32 weeks and also does not have the specialist services to look after babies needing surgery for blockage of the stomach.

Temperament: You are anxious about the delay in seeing the on call doctor. After the doctor explains that you will need to be transferred to another hospital, you demand that your husband should stay in the hospital with you as you are worried about going to another hospital although you understand this is in the baby's best interest.

Ideas: You declined the needle test for checking the chromosomes as you were anxious about the risk of miscarriage. You believe that the babies are going to be fine.

Expectations: You want the doctor to explain:

- You will have an apology for the delay and reasons explained
- If your cervix is dilated?
- Are you in labour?
- Why this has happened?
- Can labour be stopped?
- Explanations of the scan findings done on labour ward by the registrar
- Why do you need the steroid injection? How will it help the babies?
- Will you need to be delivered?
- How will they deliver you?
- Are there are any tests to find out if your waters have gone?
- Why you need to be transferred to another unit?
- Will both babies be alright?
- Does the baby with the blockage of the stomach have Downs's syndrome?
- How soon after birth can they find out if the baby has Downs's syndrome?
- How long will they need to be hospital?
- Will the twin with the problem need surgery straightaway?
- How long will she stay in hospital after her delivery?
- Can the babies survive if they were born so early?
- Can her husband stay with her in the referring hospital?

At the end there are some marks for you to award according to how well the candidate explained your questions and concerns.

Instruction for Assessors

Please read instruction to candidate and role player.

She has had a mucousy discharge overnight and she thinks she may have had a trickle of fluid loss overnight but is not entirely sure. One of the twins is known to have a double bubble appearance of stomach. This is a spontaneous Dichorionic diamniotic twin pregnancy. She has had first trimester combined screening for Downs's syndrome and both the foetuses have a low risk result of 1: 1000 and 1: 1500. Following her 20 week scan she was referred to the tertiary foetal medicine unit. The couple have declined invasive testing. She has already met with the paediatric surgeons in the tertiary unit and was advised that the baby will need to be delivered in a unit with paediatric surgical facilities.

She has had fibronectin test and this is positive. Both the babies are cephalic in presentation. The twin with the problem is the upper twin and has polyhydramnios and double bubble appearance of stomach. No other markers on scan were noted on either twin.

The candidate will need to demonstrate an understanding of the assessment of risk for preterm labour, need for in utero transfer and the procedure involved.

There are some marks on the process mark sheet for the actor to assign at the end of the station.

Record your overall clinical impression of the candidate for each domains (i.e. should this performance be pass, borderline, or a fail).

Assessment

Marking Scheme		
Patient safety:		
Pass	Borderline	Fail
Communication with patients and their relatives:		
Pass	Borderline	Fail
Information gathering:		
Pass	Borderline	Fail
Applied clinical knowledge:		
Pass	Borderline	Fail

Notes for Marking

Patient safety

- Demonstrates understanding of possible risk to mother and babies and arranges in utero transfer efficiently
- Open and honest
- No false assurance and platitudes

Communication with patients and their relatives

- Apologies for the delay in review
- Explaining reasons for delay
- Explaining reasons for in utero transfer
- Managing expectations following transfer to another hospital
- Liaising with the neonatal unit and labour ward of the recipient unit.
- Informing the on call consultant about the in utero transfer
- Explains examination findings and implications
- Reasons for antenatal steroids, tocolysis
- Summary letter with relevant findings and key issues

Information gathering

- Obtains a relevant obstetric history
- Obtains the vital information from the notes
- Obtains the patients views, expectations, and concerns

Applied clinical knowledge

- Assessment for risk of preterm labour
- Demonstrates understanding of current guidelines for management of complex twins
- Interpretation of investigations for assessment of preterm labour and preterm rupture of membranes
- Criteria for NNU admission facilities in level two unit

- Appropriate liaison for in utero transfer to level three neonatal unit with paediatric surgical facilities
- Risks to babies if born preterm
- Rational for antenatal steroids for fetal lung maturity
- Use of tocolytics for in utero transfer
- In utero transfer guidelines for the local hospital
- Involvement of the local neonatal team before transfer
- Liaising with the neonatal and obstetric teams of the receiving unit.

Notes for Candidate

Familiar with unit protocol for in utero transfer
Use of tocolytics for in utero transfer and safety of use
RCOG guidelines for antenatal steroids for fetal lung maturity
Use of fibronectin and cervical length for assessment for risk of preterm labour
Using SBAR for handover
Neonatal networks in the region

Further reading

Antenatal Corticosteroids to Reduce Neonatal Morbidity and Mortality; 2010; RCOG. https://www.rcog.org.uk/globalassets/documents/guidelines/gtg_7.pdf
Preterm labour and birth; NICE guideline [NG25] Published date: November 2015. https://www.nice.org.uk/guidance/ng25?unlid=7564651032016383455

Task 4 **Leadership: labour ward prioritization**

Instructions for Candidate

This task assesses the following clinical skills:

- Patient safety
- Communication with colleagues
- Information gathering
- Applied clinical knowledge

You are an ST-5 Doctor rostered to be the Registrar on-call for the Central Delivery Suite. You arrive promptly for the handover at 8.30 am. Your obstetric SHO and the anaesthetic registrar are already present. Your Consultant has left a message that he is running 30 minutes late due to heavy traffic. You have six labour ward midwives on duty, including the midwifery coordinator.

See Table 11.1.

You will have to decide:

1. What tasks need to be done
2. The order in which they should be done.
3. Who should be allocated to the task?

You will then discuss and justify your decisions to the assessor.

You may take notes if you wish. A writing pad has been provided. However, these notes will not carry any marks. You will only be marked on your discussion with the Assessor.

You have 10 minutes for this task (+ 2mins initial reading time).

Table 11.1 Labour ward board

Room Number	Name	Para	Gestational age	Details
1	AB	P0	40 + 2	Normal vaginal delivery at 8.05 am. Episiotomy to be sutured.
2	CD	P0	39 + 5	Normal vaginal delivery at 8.10 am. Active bleeding+++. Blood pressure 80/50mmHg.
3	EF	P1	40 + 6	Trial of vaginal birth after caesarean section. 6cm at 4.00 am and 8.00 am, contracting 1 in 5.
4	GH	P0	38 + 6	Full dilatation at 7.00 am. CTG normal. No urge to push. No descent. Nil visible.? Occipito- posterior.
5	IJ	P0	37 + 5	Not in labour. Severe PET pre-eclampsia with headache. Blood pressure 180/110mmHg.
6	KL	P1	39 + 3	6cm at 6.00 am. Bradycardia at 8.20 am, but good recovery within 4 minutes.
7	MN	P2	29 weeks	Abdominal pain. Observations normal. CTG normal.
8	OP	P1	1st postop day	Elective caesarean section, Day 2. PPH of 1.8L. No urine output for 4 hours
9	QR	P1	34 weeks	Insulin-dependent diabetes mellitus. For elective admission for antenatal steroids prior to planned caesarean section 4 days later.
10	ST	P1	34 weeks	? labour. Contracting 1 in 8.

Instructions to Assessor

Allow the candidate to read the question and decide on the management.

The candidate has up to six minutes to prepare for this station and six minutes to discuss with you. If the candidate is ready to discuss with the assessor before the six minutes, please do so. If the candidate, after 8 minutes, is still not ready for the discussion prompt the candidate initiating the discussion.

The candidate has to explain to you:

1. What needs to be done.
2. Why it needs to be done.
3. Who is going to do it.

For the mark sheet see Table 11.2.

Record your clinical impression (Pass, Borderline, or Fail) for the candidate.

Table 11.2 Labour ward board after prioritization

Room Number	Name	Para	Gestational age	Details	Category of the task	Person allocated to task	Task to be done
1	AB	P0	40 + 2	Normal vaginal delivery at 8.05 am. Episiotomy to be sutured.	3	Attending midwife in the room	No pressing urgency. Episiotomy can be sutured by the midwife as soon as convenient for both the patient and midwife.
2	CD	P0	39 + 5	Normal vaginal delivery at 8.10 am. Active bleeding+++. Blood pressure 80/50mmHg.	1	Candidate -1	As ongoing PPH with haemodynamic instability and falling BP, the first priority is treatment of PPH.
3	EF	P1	40 + 6	Trial of vaginal birth after caesarean section. 6cm at 4.00 am and 8.00 am, contracting 1 in 5.	3	SHO -1	As evidence of poor progress needs ARM for labour augmentation. Can be done by the SHO.
4	GH	P0	38 + 6	Full dilatation at 7.00 am. CTG normal. No urge to push. No descent. Nil visible.? Occipito-posterior.	2	Candidate - 2/3	As active 2nd stage has not yet commenced and CTG is normal, there is no imminent threat to the health of either the mother or child, but needs early delivery.

Room Number	Name	Para	Gestational age	Details	Category of the task	Person allocated to task	Task to be done
5	IJ	P0	37 + 5	Not in labour. Severe PET pre-eclampsia with headache. Blood pressure 180/110mmHg.	1	Candidate - 2/3	Signs of imminent eclampsia evident with immediate threat to the life of the mother.
6	KL	P1	39 + 3	6cm at 6.00 am. Bradycardia at 8.20 am, but good recovery within 4 minutes.	2	Midwifery co-ordinator -1	No immediate concerns of foetal health. Satisfactory progress. Hence midwifery coordinator can review the CTG in 15–20 minutes.
7	MN	P2	29 weeks	Abdominal pain. Observations normal. CTG normal.	3	SHO -2	No major maternal or foetal concern. Can be seen by the senior house officer after Room 3.
8	OP	P1	1st postop day	Elective caesarean section, Day 2. PPH of 1.8L. No urine output for 4 hours	2	Anaesthetist	As fluid balance is a predominant concern Anaesthetist can most effectively review this ASAP.
9	QR	P1	34 weeks	Insulin-dependent diabetes mellitus. For elective admission for antenatal steroids prior to planned caesarean section 4 days later.	4	SHO -3	No maternal or foetal concerns. Elective admission. Can be seen by SHO after Rooms 3 and 7.
10	ST	P1	34 weeks	? labour. Contracting 1 in 8.	3	Midwifery Co-ordinator—2	Possibility of pre-term labour. The Midwifery Coordinator to undertake speculum examination and foetal fibronectin after assessing Room 6.

Prioritization

Prior into entering into Room 1 the candidate should give instructions to the midwife to

- Give Labetalol to Room 5, to
- Start five minute observations

- Get the magnesium sulphate ready, and
- Insert Venflon

Whilst loading up the magnesium sulphate, the candidate could enter into Room 2. When out of Room 2 the candidate should enquire regarding Room 5's blood pressure. If now normal and headache resolved the candidate should state he/she will go into Room 4. If not will enter Room 5.

Case 1

Normal vaginal delivery at 8.05 am. Episiotomy to be sutured.

No pressing urgency. Episiotomy can be sutured by the midwife as soon as convenient for both the patient and midwife.

Case 2

Normal vaginal delivery at 8.10 am. Active bleeding+++. Blood pressure 80/50mmHg.

As ongoing PPH with haemodynamic instability and falling BP, the first priority is treatment of PPH.

Case 3

Vaginal birth after caesarean section. 6cm at 4.00 am and 8.00 am, contracting one in five.

As evidence of poor progress needs ARM for labour augmentation. Can be done by the SHO.

Case 4

Full dilatation at 7.00 am. CTG normal. No urge to push. No descent. Nil visible? Occipital posterior.

As active second stage has not yet commenced and CTG is normal there is no imminent threat to the health of either the mother or child, but needs early delivery.

Case 5

Not in labour. Severe PET pre-eclampsia with headache. Blood pressure of 180/110mmHg.

Signs of imminent eclampsia evident with immediate threat to the life of the mother.

Case 6

6cm at 6.00 am. Bradycardia at 8.20 am, but good recovery within four minutes.

No immediate concerns of foetal health. Satisfactory progress. Hence midwifery coordinator can review the CTG in 15–20 minutes.

Case 7

Abdominal pain. Observations normal. CTG normal.

No major maternal or foetal concern. Can be seen by the senior house officer after Room 3.

Case 8

Elective caesarean section, Day 2. PPH of 1.8L. No urine output.

As fluid balance is a predominant concern, anaesthetist can most effectively review this ASAP.

Case 9

Insulin-dependent diabetes mellitus. For elective admission for antenatal steroids prior to planned caesarean section four days later.

No maternal or fetal concerns. Elective admission. Can be seen by SHO after Room 3 and 7.

Case 10

In labour. Contracting 1 in 8.

Possibility of pre-term labour. The midwifery coordinator to undertake speculum examination and foetal fibronectin after assessing Room 6.

Assessment

Marking scheme		
Patient safety:		
Pass	Borderline	Fail
Communication with colleague:		
Pass	Borderline	Fail
Information gathering:		
Pass	Borderline	Fail
Applied clinical knowledge:		
Pass	Borderline	Fail

Notes for Marking

Patient safety

- Demonstrates understanding of possible risk to mother and babies and the rationale behind the chosen prioritisation

Communication with assessor

- Clear and succinct reasoning
- Inspires confidence in decision making

Information gathering

- Obtains the vital information from the notes

Applied clinical knowledge:

- Understands the different clinical problems and assesses the urgency accordingly

Notes for Candidate

This is a labour ward prioritisation station. You will be assessed for your ability to manage the delivery suite and the ability to foresee and prepare for problems.

You have up to six minutes to prepare for this station and six minutes to discuss with the Assessor. If you are ready to discuss with the assessor before the six minutes please do so.

Let the assessor know how you would be approaching the problem. My recommendation would be for categorising the urgency of the task by simply following the RCOG's own classification of the urgency of caesarean section. You should be able to describe the categories in terms of maternal and fetal health.

Urgency Definition and Category:

- Immediate threat to life of woman or foetus—category 1
- Maternal or fetal compromise, but no immediate threat to the life of woman or fetus—category 2

- No maternal or fetal compromise but requires early delivery—category 3
- At a time to suit the woman and maternity services—category 4

For each patient prepare by writing brief notes on:

1. The task to be done.
2. The urgency of the task.
3. The staff to be allocated to do the task

Do not spend more time than necessary on writing as it is more important to justify this to the Assessor. The writing pad itself would not be allocated any marks; it is what you say to the Assessor that will fetch you the necessary marks.

Exhibit your knowledge of the management of common intrapartum problems. For example, state the NICE guideline on the management of second stage of labour, other signs of imminent eclampsia, three minutes rule for bradycardia etc.

There may be some variation in the prioritisations, especially for category 2 and 3, but it is your ability to justify these decisions that matters.

Further reading

Prioritization on the labour suite, Dipanwita Kapoor, Gemma Wright, Lucy Kean, *June 2014*, Volume 24, Issue 6, Pages 157–161, *Obstetrics,Gynaecology and Reproductive medicine*. http://www.obstetrics-gynaecology-journal.com/article/S1751-7214(14)00064-5/abstract

Chapter 12 **Management of delivery**

Task 1 **Breech delivery**

Instructions for Candidate

This task assesses the following clinical skills:

- Patient safety
- Communication with patients and their relatives
- Information gathering
- Applied clinical knowledge

Rebecca Francis is a 34-year-old lady in her second pregnancy.

She has had a normal vaginal delivery two years ago.

Her pregnancy remained uneventful so far.

At 36 weeks, her midwife detected that the baby was in breech presentation and has referred her to the antenatal clinic to discuss further management.

You will then be given some information and asked questions by the examiner.

You have 10 minutes for this task (+ 2mins initial reading time).

Instructions for Assessor

Please read instruction to candidate and actor.

After the consultation with the actor patient (or in the last two minutes), tell the candidate that Rebecca underwent an unsuccessful ECV and was booked for an elective caesarean at 39 weeks.

You performed her caesarean and to your surprise, you delivered a cephalic baby by caesarean section.

What should you have done to prevent this?

What will you do next to prevent this kind of incidence? What will you explain to Rebecca?

Record your overall clinical impression of the candidate for each domain (i.e. should this performance be pass, borderline, or a fail).

Instructions for Role Player

You are Rebecca Francis, a 34-year-old mother of two-year-old Lucy. You had a straight forward pregnancy and delivery with Lucy.

You are currently 36 weeks pregnant.

You were seen by your midwife yesterday for a routine check and she found the baby to be in breech position. You were sent to the antenatal clinic and have had a scan confirming that the baby is in breech position. You were told that rest of the scan, including the baby's measurements, fluid volume around the baby and the position of the placenta are normal.

You are healthy. You do not smoke and have had no alcohol in pregnancy. Your pregnancy has progressed without any problems so far. The screening test for the baby showed low risk for Down's syndrome.

Temperament: You think you are mostly a calm, level-headed woman, but you do like to be organised and in control of things.

Ideas: You were expecting this pregnancy and delivery to be very easy and straightforward, as this is your second pregnancy.

Concerns: You want what is best for the baby, but are keen to avoid a caesarean section. Your husband's work requires him to travel a lot away from home, so you are also required to look after Lucy. You are concerned that if you need a caesarean section, then it will be difficult for you to look after Lucy and the new baby. Your husband may be able to take a few days off, but you do not have any other family support.

Expectations: You want the candidate to explain:

- What is breech presentation?
- Can anything be done to decrease the chance of the baby being breech at term?
- The ins and outs of External Cephalic Version(ECV). This is your favoured option
- What are your options regarding delivery?
- The pros and cons of vaginal breech delivery and caesarean section

At the end there are some marks for you to award according to how well the candidate communicated to you.

Assessment

Marking scheme

Patient safety:

Pass Borderline Fail

Communication with patients and their relatives:

Pass Borderline Fail

Information gathering:

Pass Borderline Fail

Applied clinical knowledge:

Pass Borderline Fail

Notes for Marking

Patient safety

- Gives options and discusses the pros and cons of each
- Involves patient in the process (e.g. encouraging them to express their ideas, or preferences)
- Negotiates a mutually agreed acceptable, safe, plan
- Open and honest about the mistake
- Offer an apology explain fully and promptly, the mistake of clinical examination and scan prior to the LSCS
- Explain mechanism in place to deal with mistakes and learn from them-incident form, audit

Communication with patients and their relatives

- Greets, introduces self and role, checks patient's name
- Consent to proceed and explains nature of interview
- Assesses patient's starting point (what the patient wants to know) and sets the agenda

- Clear organised explanation in logical sequence
- Chunks: i.e. provides information in reasonable chunks
- Checks patient's understanding
- Language (easily understood, avoids or explains jargon)
- Uses visual aids appropriately e.g. diagrams or uses analogies to aid explanation

Information gathering

- Obtains a focussed and relevant obstetric history
- Assesses the patient's main concerns and ideas

Applied clinical knowledge

- Demonstrates a sound and comprehensive evidence-based clinical knowledge
- Counsels the patient with relevant information that is factually correct.
- Makes a robust and safe management plan

Notes for Candidate

The scenario is taken from a common clinical scenario of our daily practice. It not only assesses the process of communication but also assesses the content of the knowledge given to the patient. It is important *how* you provide the information to the patient.

Make yourself aware of the success rate of ECV in your unit. Be familiar with incident reporting and mechanisms for wider learning from mistakes.

Practice this scenario with one of your friends who can act as a role player and ask another friend to provide you with feedback.

What to include in counselling

Explanation of presentation

- Breech means that your baby is lying bottom first or feet first in the womb instead of in the usual head first position
- In early pregnancy breech is very common. As pregnancy continues, a baby usually turns by itself into the head first position. Between 37 and 42 weeks (term), most babies are lying head first, ready to be born
- There is higher perinatal mortality and morbidity with breech than cephalic presentation, due principally to prematurity, congenital malformations, and birth asphyxia or trauma
- However, breech presentation, whatever the mode of delivery, is associated with increased risk of subsequent handicap

Option— ECV

- Vaginal breech birth is more complicated than normal birth.
- Advise trying to turn your baby to a head-first position. This technique is called external cephalic version (ECV). This is when gentle pressure is applied on your abdomen which helps the baby turn a somersault in the womb to lie head first
- ECV increases the likelihood of having a vaginal birth
- ECV is usually tried after 36 weeks
- ECV is successful for about half of all women (50%)
- should give information about your own individual chance of success

- Relaxing the muscles of the womb with medication during an ECV is likely to improve the chance of success. This medication will not affect the baby
- ECV is generally safe and does not cause labour to begin. The baby's heart will be monitored before and after the ECV
- Like any medical procedure, complications can sometimes occur. Rarely emergency caesarean section immediately after an ECV because of bleeding from the placenta and/or changes in the baby's heartbeat
- ECV can be uncomfortable
- If the baby does not want to turn, we will discuss your options for birth

Option—planned caesarean section

- Women should be informed that planned caesarean section carries a reduced perinatal mortality and early neonatal morbidity for babies with a breech presentation at term compared with planned vaginal birth
- Women should be advised that planned caesarean section for breech presentation carries a small increase in serious immediate complications for them compared with planned vaginal birth

Option—vaginal breech delivery

- Mentions the Term Breech trial
- Mentions the Dutch trial
- The Royal College of Obstetricians and Gynaecologists currently recommends that caesarean delivery is the safest mode of delivery for the baby when in a breech position
- If for vaginal breech—delivery in hospital
- Strict criteria to be followed
- Experienced accoucher to be available

Caesarean section—cephalic presentation

- Apologies
- Should have performed a scan to check presentation before caesarean
- You will do an incident report
- Confirm guideline exists to check presentation by ultrasound prior to caesarean section
- Audit the implementation of the guideline

Further reading

RCOG, External Cephalic Version and reducing the incidence of Breech presentation,Guideline No. 20a. https://www.rcog.org.uk/globalassets/documents/guidelines/gt20aexternalcephalicversion.pdf

RCOG, the Management of Breech Presentation, Guideline No. 20b https://www.rcog.org.uk/globalassets/documents/guidelines/gtg-no-20b-breech-presentation.pdf

Task 2 **Caesarean section**

Instructions for Candidate

This task assesses the following clinical skills:

- Patient safety
- Communication with colleagues
- Applied clinical knowledge

You are the registrar on duty and have just finished a caesarean section performed at full dilatation. You are sitting with your senior SHO who is keen on discussing this further. Your SHO has the following questions:

- Was this avoidable?
- What are the associated maternal and neonatal risk?
- What is the optimal management for CS at full dilatation?

You are expected to answer trainee's questions evolving around the points mentioned in discussion and demonstrate your knowledge on the subject.

You have 10 minutes for this task (+ 2mins initial reading time).

Instructions for Assessor

You will act as the junior colleague. This conversation is going to be among two professionals where the ST5 should demonstrate knowledge about the questions asked. You are keen to know your registrar's experience about it. Ask your registrar the following questions:

- I've read that the incidence of C-section at full dilatation is rising. What is your experience about it and what reasons do you think are contributing to this high rate?
- How can we avoid a second stage C section?
- What are the risks associated with the second stage CS when compared with first stage CS and instrumental delivery?
- What is the evidence with regards to management options for CS at full dilatation?
- Are there any specific training programmes that are available to address this situation?

Record your overall clinical impression of the candidate for each domain (e.g. should this performance be pass, borderline, or a fail).

Assessment

Marking scheme

Patient safety:

Pass Borderline Fail

Communication with colleagues:

Pass Borderline Fail

Applied clinical knowledge:

Pass Borderline Fail

Notes for Marking

Patient safety

- Demonstrates understanding of principles of safe surgery
- Demonstrates understanding of consent
- Recognises limits of their clinical abilities and demonstrates an understanding of when to call for help and involve senior colleagues and other disciplines
- Demonstrates understanding of lack of evidence on the optimal management options
- Emphasises on adequate training before embarking on expected complicated surgery

Communication with the colleague

- Ability to communicate clearly and with an ordered approach e.g. pre-operative, intra-operative, post-operative concerns
- Demonstrates ability to teach appropriate skills to other colleagues in a logical and coherent manner with recognition of the learner, environment and resources available

Applied clinical knowledge

- Demonstrates a sound and comprehensive evidence-based clinical knowledge using the information mentioned. Demonstrates understanding of essential pre-operative assessment. Knowledge in relation to obstetric surgery including techniques and the risks and benefits of procedures

Notes for Candidate

Practice this scenario with one of your friends who can act as a role player and ask another friend to provide you with feedback.

Was this avoidable?

- Careful assessment of each case individually with regards to suitability of instrumental delivery
- Involving consultant in decision making and performing a rotational or suspected difficult instrumental delivery, may avoid the surgery
- Vaginal re-assessment just prior to beginning the procedure

Reasons of increasing incidence of C section at full dilatation

- Increasing rates of failed operative vaginal delivery
- Reduced attempts at vaginal delivery
- Fewer working hours of junior doctors resulting in less exposure and confidence in performing instrumental deliveries

Associated maternal, foetal and neonatal risks

CS has a higher rate of complications as compared to vaginal birth. CS at full dilatation poses additional risks over the background risk caesarean section.

Maternal:

- Double risk of intraoperative trauma at full dilatation as compared to first stage CS i.e. laceration to bladder/bowel, extension of uterine incision, vaginal trauma due to failed instrumental delivery etc.
- Increased risk of haemorrhage at full dilatation as compared to first stage CS

- Psychological morbidity e.g. fear of future childbirth, dyspareunia etc.
- Long term morbidity in terms of urinary incontinence

Neonatal:

- Overall severe trauma is low in association with CS, both full dilatation as well as first stage
- Trauma can be associated with attempts of failed instrumental delivery e.g. bruising
- More admissions to SCBU due to lower Apgar scores and blood pH compared to babies born vaginally
- Babies born by CS at full dilatation are 1.5 times more likely to have perinatal asphyxia than those born by CS during first stage

Optimal management

No national guidelines addressing specifically the management of CS at full dilatation. Optimal management is based on good practice and clinical experience.

Incision:

- Higher incision in the uterus to avoid risk of incising bladder, vagina, cervix
- Lower incisions are at higher risk of tearing and more difficult to repair

Deeply engaged presenting part:

Disimpacting the foetus can be problematic
Any ongoing oxytocin infusion must be stopped
Disimpaction is best tried in between contractions, no evidence in support of using uterine relaxants with an added risk of PPH

The following techniques can be tried but none is supported by evidence over the other:

- Push method from vagina
- Use of non-dominant hand to aid flexion and rotation of the head while exerting steady pressure upwards on the foetal head
- Patwardhan's method: delivery of both foetal shoulders through the incision followed by the trunk, breech, and then finally lifting the head out of the pelvis

All these techniques are associated with increased risk of extension of uterine incision
Use of devices:

Foetal disimpacting system
C-snorkel

No strong studies present to support use of either of these methods.

Training:

No formal training programmes, need to develop such programmes
Involvement of consultant in decision making and presence at the time of surgery may help
Place of structured protocols
Skills and training on simulated models can help reduce the force used at the time of delivery

Further reading

RCOG, *The Obstetrician and Gynaecologist*, Caesarean section at full dilatation: incidence, impact and current management, Volume 16, Issue 3, pages 199–205, July 2014.

Task 3 **Shoulder dystocia**

Instructions for Candidate

This task assesses the following clinical skills:

- Patient safety
- Communication with colleagues
- Applied clinical knowledge

You are on call on the delivery suite and had to attend the emergency buzzer when Louise Reeve was delivering her first baby. She has Type II diabetes and her BMI is 48. Her blood sugars were not very well controlled in pregnancy and she had induction of labour at 37 weeks of pregnancy. Labour progressed slowly, she started pushing after your rounds at 09.00 pm. When you arrived in the room, baby's head was delivered but there was difficulty with the shoulders. You took the lead and delivered the baby after several maneuvers. Taking the same scenario as an example, you are expected to demonstrate the maneuvers of shoulder dystocia on this station.

There is no role player on this station. You will demonstrate the skills to the examiner on a mannequin.

You have 10 minutes for this task (+ 2mins initial reading time).

Instructions for Assessor

This is a practical skills station and the candidate should demonstrate their ability to deal with emergencies by identifying the potential risks and the urgency of the situation. Using the mannequin, they should demonstrate the manoeuvres while simultaneously communicating and managing the patient.

Use the criteria mentioned in the next section in the marking scheme to ensure an up-to mark teaching session.

Assessment

Marking scheme

Patient safety:

Pass	Borderline	Fail

Communication with colleagues:

Pass	Borderline	Fail

Applied clinical knowledge:

Pass	Borderline	Fail

Notes for Marking

Patient safety

- The candidate must include following points of safety and quality:
  - Demonstrates ability to identify risk factors.
  - When to involve a consultant
  - Demonstrates understanding of clinical governance and risk management (incident reporting)

- Importance of adequate training in the form of skills and drills
- Highlights importance of adherence to policies and procedures
- Highlights importance of meticulous documentation (names of staff, timings of manoeuvres, side of foetal back, which shoulder was posterior)

Communication with colleagues

- Demonstrates ability to communicate with the patient, relatives, team members and multidisciplinary team in a logical and coherent manner
- Also emphasises importance of team work, call for help, roles assigning to various team members during manoeuvres etc.
- The candidate should demonstrate all or most of the following teamwork skills:
  - Asks for help
  - Transmits requests directly to individual team members
  - Shows good leadership skills, and delegates tasks
  - Provides positive feedback to the team at the end

During the practical skills session, the candidate must demonstrate their ability to:

- Identify risk factors
- Staff and patient's debriefing
- Ensuring patient understanding and encouraging questions

Provides a clear and relevant explanation of events at the end, adapted to the patient's knowledge and presented in a logical sequence

Applied clinical knowledge

- The candidate should be able to demonstrate the awareness of dealing with an emergency and the reason behind the shoulder dystocia. They should demonstrate their ability to apply all manoeuvres keeping in view the main cause of shoulder dystocia i.e. should concentrate on reducing the bisacromial diameter of shoulders as well as widening the pelvis. They should be able to demonstrate awareness of the risks of shoulder dystocia and the manoeuvres to both mother and foetus. The manoeuvres should be demonstrated using HELPPER pneumonic. Technical skills that they should demonstrate should include all or most of the following:
  - Makes diagnosis of shoulder dystocia and inform all the team
  - Requests McRobert's manoeuvre
  - Requests suprapubic pressure
  - Delivers using an appropriately applied internal manoeuvre (rotation of anterior shoulder, rotation of posterior shoulder, extraction of posterior arm)

Notes for Candidate

The scenario is about one of the obstetric emergencies. It not only assesses the process of communication, your emergency skills and the content of the knowledge around the subject. It's important how you demonstrate the skills practically instead of saying and not doing.

Practice this scenario with one of your friends who can act as a role player and ask another friend to provide you with feedback.

Further reading

RCOG, Clinical Green top guideline on Shoulder Dystocia RCOG: guideline number 42. https://www.rcog.org.uk/globalassets/documents/guidelines/gtg_42.pdf

Chapter 13 **Puerperal problems**

Task 1 **Post-natal depression**

Instructions for candidate

This task assesses the following clinical skills:

- Patient safety
- Communication with patients and their relatives
- Information gathering
- Applied clinical knowledge

Anna Polanska, a 34-year-old woman, is ten days postpartum. Anna underwent induction of labour for reduced foetal movements and small for gestational age and had a ventouse delivery complicated by a third degree tear. She was discharged home, but her baby is on the neonatal unit.

She has been referred by her GP as Anna is feeling very tearful over the last few days and is low in mood. She has not been sleeping well and has intrusive thoughts.

You are the registrar on call on the delivery suite and have been asked to assess Anna.

Your task is to:

- Take an appropriate history
- Organize the immediate management

You have 10 minutes for this task (+ 2mins initial reading time).

Instruction for Assessor

Please read instruction to candidate and role player.

This clinical assessment task is to assess the communication skills of the candidates and assess their understanding of the factors predisposing to postnatal depression. It also assesses if the candidates are aware of the next steps of management in such a case.

Record your overall clinical impression of the candidate for each domain (i.e. should this performance be pass, borderline, or a fail).

For marking the impression on communication skills, please consult the role player.

Instructions for Role Player

You are Anna Polanska, a 34-year-old, asylum seeker and have been in the UK for the last 18 months. You have no support from your ex-partner and do not have any family in the UK.

You gave birth to your first child ten days ago.

You booked late in this pregnancy as you were contemplating terminating the pregnancy but found out on your first scan that you were already 24 weeks pregnant and so decided to continue with the pregnancy. You were told your blood tests were normal at booking.

Your community midwife has been on sick leave and you have no money to attend hospital visits. You have not attended a few of your antenatal clinic appointments. You smoke up to 20 cigarettes per day. On scans the baby was found to be smaller than average and there was excessive fluid around the baby. You had scans again at 28, 32, and 36 weeks. You were told that there was increased amount of fluid around the baby and that your baby was smaller than expected. You were not surprised as both you and your ex-partner are small people. You had a diabetes test and that was normal.

Labour was induced at 39 weeks of gestation. You had a prolonged labour lasting 36 hours after they started induction. You had declined an epidural in labour and used gas and air. You needed to be helped with the suction cup to deliver your baby as despite your best efforts, there was no progress after you were fully dilated. You had a bad tear going to the back passage. Your baby weighed 2.6kg. Since birth your baby has been grunting and was examined by the baby doctors. He needed help to breathe. You have been told that your baby has a heart defect and a connection exists between his wind and food pipe and will need surgery for this. You are upset as you cannot understand why this was not picked up on so many scans.

Your baby was born ten days ago and is on the neonatal unit in the same hospital.

For the last four to five days you are feeling unwell. You are very tearful and feel very low in mood. You have intrusive thoughts and feel worthless and depressed. You do not have suicidal thoughts or thoughts to harm the baby. You want your baby with you and are very keen to breastfeed.

You do not have any past history of any medical problems or any mental health issues.

Temperament: You are tearful and tired. You feel guilty and are blaming yourself for the outcome of the baby.

Ideas: You were expecting the delivery to be straightforward.

Concerns: You want the best care for the baby. You are also angry that the problem with the baby's heart was not diagnosed on scans. You are keen to breast fed the baby. You are not keen to take any medications for your symptoms of low mood and tearfulness as you think this will be passed on to the baby. You think the medications will cause harm to the baby.

You had been experiencing significant pain from the perineal tear.

Expectations: You want a full explanation of what is going to happen to the baby. You expect that the doctor will help you to provide support and confidence so that you can look after the baby. You do not want to harm your baby.

Assessment

Marking scheme:

Patient safety:

Pass	Borderline	Fail

Communication with patients and their relatives:

Pass	Borderline	Fail

Information gathering:

Pass	Borderline	Fail

Applied clinical knowledge:

Pass	Borderline	Fail

Notes for Marking

Patient safety

- Assesses patient's main concerns
- Gives options and discusses the pros and cons of antidepressant medications whilst breastfeeding

- Involves patient in the process (e.g. encouraging them to express their ideas, or preferences)
- Negotiates a mutually agreed, acceptable, and safe management plan

Communication with patients and their relatives

- Greets, introduces self and role, checks patient's name
- Consent to proceed and explains nature of interview
- Assesses patient's starting point (what the patient wants to know) and sets the agenda
- Clear organized explanation in logical sequence
- Chunks: i.e. provides information in reasonable chunks
- Checks patient's understanding.
- Language (easily understood, avoids or explains jargon)
- Uses visual aids appropriately e.g. diagrams or uses analogies to aid explanation
- Deal with anger and concerns raised by the patient

Information gathering

- Obtains a relevant obstetric history
- Obtains views, expectations, and concerns regarding both herself and the baby

Applied clinical knowledge

- Demonstrates a sound and comprehensive evidence-based clinical knowledge
- Counsels the patient with relevant information about limitations of antenatal screening
- Recognizes risk factors and symptoms of postnatal depression
- Discusses options for treatment
- Aware of the predisposing factors for post-natal depression-Asylum seeker, no family, baby in neonatal unit, financial constraints. Feeling of guilt

Notes for Candidate

- Assessment of risk factors for postnatal depression
- Asylum seeker
- Poor social support
- Traumatic birth experience
- Neonatal concerns
- Detailed history and recognize symptoms of depression and anxiety
- Low mood
- Tearful
- Intrusive thoughts
- Insomnia
- Loss of appetite
- Appropriate assessment and referral
- Awareness about the emotional changes in childbirth
- 10% of women develop depressive symptoms postnatally
- Involve perinatal mental health team in management
- Evidence-based discussion about safety of medications with breastfeeding
- Offer psychological support
- Explain risks to the mother if not treated or worsening of symptoms
- Explain risk factors, implications of clinical symptoms and prognosis

- Ensure appropriate follow up
- Inform GP and community midwife
- Unexpected neonatal concerns
- Limitations of antenatal screening
- Cardiac screening even with extended views (outflow tracts) up to 50% antenatal diagnosis
- Tracheoesophageal fistula may not be diagnosed antenatally as foetal stomach may be present
- Risk factors on scan including small for gestational age and polyhydramnios
- Appropriate counselling for common causes of scan findings including chromosomal, genetic, structural abnormalities
- Involve neonatal team during discussions
- Feedback to antenatal screening co-ordinator
- Complete an incident form and Duty of Candour

Further reading

Antenatal and postnatal mental health: clinical management and service guidance Clinical guideline [CG192] Published date: December 2014 Last updated: June 2015, National institute for Health and care excellence. https://www.nice.org.uk/guidance/CG192

Management of Women with Mental Health Issues during Pregnancy and the Postnatal Period, Good practice, No 14, June 2011. https://www.rcog.org.uk/globalassets/documents/guidelines/managementwomenmentalhealthgoodpractice14.pdf

Task 2 **Thrombo-embolism**

Instructions for Candidate

This task assesses the following clinical skills:

- Patient safety
- Communication with patients and their relatives
- Information gathering
- Applied clinical knowledge

You are the registrar on call and have been asked by your SHO to review a patient on the post-natal ward who she is concerned about.

Mrs Susan Morris is a 28-year-old lady who is day four post-partum. She is complaining of difficulty in breathing and some chest pain.

She had an uncomplicated emergency caesarean section for failure to progress with an EBL of 800mL.

You have access to her notes, observation chart and drug chart. You will be provided with the examination findings on enquiry only.

Your task is to:

- Take a history (examination findings will be given to you by the examiner)
- Organize necessary investigations
- Interpret the results
- Initiate the management
- Justify your answers

You have 10 minutes for this task (+ 2mins initial reading time).

Instructions for Assessor

This patient has a Pulmonary Embolism. When asked please provide the following examination findings to the candidate.

Observations:

HR—106
BP—110/82
RR—18
Sats—95%
Temperatute—36.5
O/E-BMI—32
Capillary refill time—>3 seconds
Per Abdomen—soft, mild tenderness over the Caesarean section scar
Wound Healing—bowel sounds present
Chest examination—good air entry bilaterally, no wheeze or crackles, normal heart sounds, no added sounds or murmur

Ask about the next set of investigations. Tell compression Duplex Ultrasound of deep veins is negative and chest X-ray looks suspicious.

A good candidate should opt for CTPA.

Record your overall clinical impression of the candidate for each domain (i.e. should this performance be pass, borderline, or a fail).

Instructions for Role Player

You are Susan Morris, 28-years-old who had a caesarean section four days ago.

This is your first child and the caesarean was done as you got stuck at 5cm dilated. You have remained in hospital since as your baby is having iv antibiotics.

You have found it quite painful to walk around so have spent most of your time in bed, your partner and other family members have been doing a lot for you so that you don't have to move.

You were given some stockings to wear, but it's very hot on the post-natal ward and so you have taken them off.

For the past 12 hours you have felt increasingly short of breath and complain of a central chest pain. The pain is quite sharp and you are confused as to why you are feeling worse than you did straight after the caesarean.

Assessment

Marking scheme

Patient safety:

Pass Borderline Fail

Communication with patients and their relatives:

Pass Borderline Fail

Information gathering:

Pass Borderline Fail

Applied clinical knowledge:

Pass Borderline Fail

Notes for Marking

Patient safety

- Assesses the patient's main concerns and ideas
- Gives options and discusses the pros and cons of different management plans
- Discusses possible complications and measures to reduce them
- Involves patient in the process (e.g. encouraging them to express their ideas, or preferences)
- Negotiates a mutually agreed acceptable, safe, plan
- Open and honest about procedure and possible complications
- Explains mechanism in place to deal with complications and learn from complications

Communication with patients and their relatives

- Greets, introduces self and role, checks patient's name
- Consent to proceed and explains nature of interview
- Assesses patient's starting point (what the patient wants to know) and sets the agenda
- Clear organized explanation in logical sequence

- Chunks: i.e. provides information in reasonable chunks
- Checks patient's understanding
- Language (easily understood, avoids or explains jargon)
- Uses visual aids appropriately e.g. diagrams or uses analogies to aid explanation
- Presents a clear and succinct history to the assessor

Information gathering

- Obtains a relevant Obstetric history
- Obtains a focused history in keeping with the emergency situation

Applied clinical knowledge

- Demonstrates a sound and comprehensive evidence-based clinical knowledge as discussed under the following heading

Notes for Candidate

Any woman with symptoms and/or signs of VTE should have objective testing performed expeditiously and treatment with low-molecular-weight heparin (LMWH) until the diagnosis is excluded by objective testing, unless treatment is strongly contraindicated. LMWH should be given in doses titrated against the woman's booking or early pregnancy weight. There is insufficient evidence to recommend whether the dose of LMWH should be given once daily or in two divided doses.

In women with suspected PE who also have symptoms and signs of DVT, compression duplex ultrasound should be performed. If compression ultrasonography confirms the presence of DVT, no further investigation is necessary and treatment for VTE should continue.

In women with suspected PE without symptoms and signs of DVT, a ventilation/perfusion (V/Q) lung scan or a computerized tomography pulmonary angiogram (CTPA) should be performed. When the chest X-ray is abnormal and there is a clinical suspicion of PE, CTPA should be performed in preference to a V/Q scan.

Alternative or repeat testing should be carried out where V/Q scan or CTPA is normal but the clinical suspicion of PE remains. Anticoagulant treatment should be continued until PE is definitively excluded.

Women with suspected PE should be advised that, compared with CTPA, V/Q scanning may carry a slightly increased risk of childhood cancer but is associated with a lower risk of maternal breast cancer; in both situations, the absolute risk is very small.

D-dimer testing should **not** be performed in the investigation of acute VTE in pregnancy. Before anticoagulant therapy is commenced, blood should be taken for a full blood count, coagulation screen, urea and electrolytes, and liver function tests. Performing a thrombophilia screen prior to therapy is not recommended.

Obstetric patients who are postoperative and receiving unfractionated heparin should have platelet count monitoring performed every two to three days from days four to 14 or until heparin is stopped.

Therapeutic anticoagulant therapy should be continued for the duration of the pregnancy and for at least six weeks postnatally and until at least three months of treatment has been given in total. Before discontinuing treatment, the continuing risk of thrombosis should be assessed.

Women should be offered a choice of LMWH or oral anticoagulant for postnatal therapy after discussion about the need for regular blood tests for monitoring of warfarin, particularly during the first ten days of treatment. Postpartum warfarin should be avoided until at least the fifth day and for longer in women at increased risk of postpartum haemorrhage.

Women should be advised that neither heparin (unfractionated or LMWH) nor warfarin is contraindicated in breastfeeding.

Further reading

RCOG Green-top Guideline No. 37b 2 of 32 © Royal College of Obstetricians and Gynaecologists. https://www.rcog.org.uk/globalassets/documents/guidelines/gtg-37b.pdf

Catherine Nelson-Piercy, *Handbook of obstetric medicine* 5th ed, 2015. CRC Press.

Task 3 **Post-CS Sepsis**

Instructions for Candidate

This task assesses the following clinical skills:

- Patient safety
- Communication with colleagues
- Applied clinical knowledge

You presented a case in your departmental morbidity and mortality meeting. This lady was readmitted with post-operative sepsis ten days after an emergency Caesarean section. She was admitted really ill and had remained in critical care for five days. She had to remain in the hospital for ten days before she could be discharged back home. Her husband had been very difficult in the initial days and was convinced that if his wife dies because of the sepsis, this will be hospital's fault to have given her this nasty infection. After you have presented the case, your consultant asks you following questions:

How would you identify risks contributing to post-caesarean sepsis?
How would you analyse and evaluate the situation?
What will you do to avoid this to happen in the future?

You will be asked these questions by the examiner on the station.

You have 10 minutes for this task (+ 2mins initial reading time).

Instructions for Assessor

This is a risk management station and the candidate should demonstrate their understanding of risk management process and the RADICAL framework. They should cover most or all of the elements mentioned under every question.

Record your overall clinical impression of the candidate for each domain (i.e. should this performance be pass, borderline, or a fail).

Assessment

Marking scheme

Patient safety:

Pass	Borderline	Fail

Communication with colleagues:

Pass	Borderline	Fail

Applied clinical knowledge:

Pass	Borderline	Fail

Notes for Marking

Patient safety and quality

- Demonstrates awareness of the systems in place that ensure patient safety and quality of services delivered e.g. policies and procedures

- Open and honest in sharing the results of the risk assessment with colleagues and the patient by answering Question 3

Communication with colleagues

- Demonstrates the understanding the importance of channels of communication while dealing with risk management e.g. reports, statements, incident reporting, complaints

Applied clinical knowledge

- Demonstrates a sound and comprehensive knowledge on the process of risk management and RADICAL framework. Including as many points as possible as mentioned previously

Notes for Candidate

In this station you will be given a set of patient's records to look at. It is important you develop the skills of case note reviewing to look at the care received by the patient.

How would you identify risks contributing to sepsis?

This question should lead the candidate to demonstrate their understanding of how risks are identified rather than what the risks in these patients were. They should be able to acknowledge that in this case it will be retrospective risk identification and can be done using the following resources:

- Review notes
- Talk to staff involved
- Request reports
- Check documentations to identify all contributing risk factors (use fishbone model)
- Check if incident reports were filled
- Check if any complaint was raised and what was done about it

How would you analyse and evaluate the situation?

- Identify incident and take decisions to investigate
- Select members of investigation team
- Gather data (such as records, interviews, protocols) and relevant physical items
- Determine the chronology of the incident
- Identify care delivery problems (unsafe acts e.g. failure to act or incorrect decision)
- Identify contributory factors (such as inadequate training, lack of supervision)
- Devise an action plan

What will you do to avoid this to happen in the future?

Share lessons learnt from risk identification. Raise awareness. Channels that can be used for sharing the lessons are:

- Multidisciplinary team meetings
- Ward meetings
- Safety alerts
- News letters
- Intranet
- Educational meetings

Further reading

Improving patient safety: risk management for maternity and gynaecology Clinical Governance Advice No. 2, September 2009. https://www.rcog.org.uk/globalassets/documents/guidelines/clinical-governance-advice/cga2improvingpatientsafety2009.pdf

Presenting information on risk, Clinical Governance Advice No. 7, December 2008. https://www.rcog.org.uk/globalassets/documents/guidelines/clinical-governance-advice/cga7-15072010.pdf

Task 4 **Sepsis**

Instructions for Candidate

This task assesses the following clinical skills:

- Patient safety
- Communication with colleagues
- Information gathering
- Applied clinical knowledge

You are the registrar on call for a labour ward.

The labour ward co-ordinator requests you to take a telephone call from an anxious midwife in the community looking after a post-natal patient.

The first clinical scenario

An 18-year-old caucasian woman has had a normal vaginal delivery four days ago. She is complaining of worsening dysuria and supra-pubic pain since the delivery. Apart from one episode of cystitis at 32 weeks the antenatal period was uneventful. She is systemically well. Observations are all normal.

Please conduct the telephone conversation with the midwife. The assessor will assume the role of the midwife.

You have 4 minutes for this task.

The midwifery co-ordinator interrupts the telephone conversation and requests you to cut it short and urgently attend to another post-natal lady brought in via ambulance. The examiner will ask you specific questions regarding your approach to this clinical scenario.

The second scenario

A 42-year-old Afro-Caribbean woman with a BMI of 43 has been brought in via ambulance. She has had a caesarean section in labour for failure to progress at 8cm following prolonged rupture of membranes of more than 48 hours. She is conscious and oriented but quiet and withdrawn. Her observations are: Pulse rate 110. Blood pressure 90/60. Temperature: 38.4°C.

On examination the caesarean section wound looks infected with pus evident on pressure of the wound. The lochia is normal.

The assessor will ask you a series of questions regarding the management. You have 5 minutes to answer 10 questions.

In total you have 10 minutes for this task (+ 2mins initial reading time).

Instructions for Assessor

This clinical assessment task station expects a good deal more input from the assessor. The assessor is expected to steer the conversation along the suggested format—especially so for the second scenario.

Where there is significant deviation from the suggested format, gently bring back the conversation to the suggested format. Do not penalize for variation in the sequence of the questions asked. Allow for considerable variation in the language used as long as the meaning has been conveyed.

First scenario

The outline of the telephone conversation is presented as an aid to ensure that the conversation proceeds along the following lines:

Question from doctor/candidate: Hello, I am Dr X covering the labour ward. I have been asked to speak to you by a labour ward co-ordinator. How can I help you?

Answer from midwife: I am a community midwife. My patient, Ms. Y, is an 18-year-old caucasian woman has had a normal vaginal delivery four days ago. She is complaining of worsening dysuria and supra-pubic pain since the delivery. My concern is whether this could be a case of puerperal sepsis?

Question from doctor: Sure. It is possible; however I need more information first. Please can you answer a few questions regarding the patient?

Answer from midwife: Yes.

Question from doctor: Has the patient got any risk factors for puerperal sepsis? For example: Group A streptococcal colonization, recurrent UTI, obesity, anaemia, history of pelvic infections, prolonged rupture of membranes, is from black or ethnic minority groups?

Answer from midwife: Apart from one episode of cystitis at 32 weeks which responded well to antibiotics, her pregnancy has been uneventful. She has had no further episodes of UTI's.

Question from doctor: How is the patient? Is she conscious and otherwise well?

Answer from midwife: Yes, she is well, observations are stable (normal) getting about her everyday activities and taking good care of herself and the baby.

Question from doctor: Does she have any flank pain, diarrhoea or vomiting, rash, vaginal discharge, or abnormal lochia?

Answer from midwife: No. She has none of the described symptoms.

Question from doctor: Has the patient got any localising signs of sepsis? For example: breast, chest, episiotomy wound, throat etc.

Answer from midwife: No, her breasts are normal. Her chest is clear and the episiotomy wound is healing well.

Question from doctor: Have you checked her urine dipstick?

Answer from midwife: Yes I have. It shows +++ leukocytes, ++ protein, + blood and nitrites positive.

Question from doctor: It is likely that her problem is UTI viz lower urinary tract infection/cystitis. What do you think?

Answer from midwife: Yes I suspect so. What should I do now?

Response from doctor: Please send a mid-stream sample of urine for culture and sensitivity. Advise adequate hydration, avoidance of bubble baths, and for pain relief I would suggest Paracetamol and not NSAID's.

Question from midwife: What antibiotic would be appropriate or how should I treat her?

Answer from doctor: Trimethoprim is appropriate as it is uncomplicated lower urinary tract infection. It is safe in breast feeding women and can be given as a three day oral course. She could get this either from her GP or from the hospital by prescription.

Question from midwife: Any follow up arrangements? Do I need to watch out for anything at all?

Answer from doctor: Yes. Worsening symptoms, no response to antibiotics in 48 hours, clinical signs of sepsis, pyrexia more than 38°, sustained tachycardia, breathlessness, abdominal or chest pain and generally unwell patient are all signs of deterioration. Please refer urgently if you notice any of these signs or symptoms.

I will have to leave now. Thank you.

Second scenario

A 42-year-old Afro-Caribbean woman with a BMI of 43 has been brought in via ambulance. She has had a caesarean section in labour for failure to progress at 8cm following prolonged rupture of membranes of more than 48 hours. She is conscious and oriented but quiet and withdrawn. Her observations are: Pulse rate 110. Blood pressure 90/60. Temperature: 38.4°C.

On examination the caesarean section wound looks infected with pus evident on pressure of the wound. The lochia is normal.

Question from the assessor: What is your preliminary diagnosis?

Answer from the candidate: Severe puerperal sepsis. Allow for sepsis.

Question: What risk factors in the picture make you suspect this diagnosis?

Answer: Obesity, black ethnic minority, caesarean section, prolonged rupture of membranes and clinical signs of hypotension, tachycardia and pyrexia.

Question: What is the difference between sepsis, severe sepsis and septic shock?

Answer: Sepsis is defined as infection plus systemic manifestations of infection. Severe sepsis is defined as sepsis plus sepsis induced organ dysfunction or tissue hypoperfusion. Septic shock is defined as the persistence of hypoperfusion despite adequate fluid replacement therapy.

Question: What are the immediate measures that you would undertake?

Answer: The immediate measures would be the Sepsis 6 Care Bundle which has to be performed within six hours of suspicion of severe sepsis:

(1) Obtain blood cultures prior to antibiotic administration
(2) Administer broad spectrum antibiotics within one hour of recognition of severe sepsis
(3) Measure serum lactate
(4) As this patient has got hypotension I would deliver an initial bolus of crystalloid minimum of 20mls per kg body weight
(5) I would commence Paracetamol for the pyrexia

Question: What is your preferred antibiotic and why?

Answer: The preferred antibiotic would be Vancomycin and Clindamycin which would be empirical antibiotics to use as per the RCOG Guidelines for caesarean section wound infection.

These are broad spectrum antibiotics and are given intravenously within an hour of suspicion of severe sepsis.

These antibiotics are preferred as the common causative organisms for caesarean section wound infection are streptococci and staphylococci—either methicillin resistant or sensitive. Clindamycin covers most streptococci and staphylococci. It is not nephrotoxic and switches off the production of exotoxins and therefore does offer broad spectrum cover.

Question: How would you monitor women with suspected sepsis?

Answer: Women with suspected sepsis should have regular observations of all their vital signs at least every half hour including temperature, pulse rate, blood pressure, and respiratory rate.

This should be recorded on a MEOWS chart (which is Modified Early Obstetric Warning Score Chart).

Question: Are there any infection control issues to be addressed?

Answer: Yes, the woman should be isolated in a single room with en suite facilities to reduce the risk of transmission of infection, as numerous streptococcal outbreaks have occurred in maternity units with shared toilet and shower facilities.

Health care workers such as doctors, midwives, nurses, anaesthetists, and the wound care team should wear personal protective equipment including disposable gloves and aprons when in contact with the woman, equipment and the surroundings.

Breaks in the skin of the woman or the carer must be covered with a waterproof dressing.

Fluid repellent surgical masks with visors must be used at operative debridement where droplet spread is possible.

Visitors should be offered suitable information and relevant personal protective equipment whilst the woman is isolated.

Question: Are there any neonatal issues to be addressed?

Answer: Women with puerperal sepsis should be aware that the baby is especially at risk of streptococcal or staphylococcal infection during birth and during breast feeding.

The umbilical area should be examined and a paediatrician consulted in the event of puerperal sepsis.

Antimicrobial prophylaxis would be appropriate as routine to neonates of mothers with GAS (Group A streptococci) infection.

Question: Is there a role for surgery?

Answer: Wound exploration or debridement should be undertaken if there is no response to antibiotics in 48 hours.

Question: Any multi-disciplinary input that you would seek?

Answer: I would obtain the input from (1) my senior colleague—consultant (2) the microbiologist, and (3) the anaesthetist/intensivist to monitor the haemodynamic status of the patient. Complete an incident form as readmission following caesarean section.

Record your overall clinical impression (Pass/Borderline/Fail) of the candidate for each of the domain.

Assessment

Marking scheme		
Patient safety:		
Pass	Borderline	Fail
Communication with colleague:		
Pass	Borderline	Fail
Information gathering:		
Pass	Borderline	Fail
Applied clinical knowledge:		
Pass	Borderline	Fail

Notes for Marking

Patient safety

- Awareness of neonatal and maternal complications and polices to prevent such complications
- Discusses infection control issues and measures to reduce them
- Provides support to the community midwife and provides clear instruction when to refer or contact
- Ensures process is place to discuss readmission with sepsis in place

Communication with colleagues

- Multi-disciplinary working is integral to good patient care. This station tests the communication skills of the candidate with allied medical staff as opposed to patients
- This station is also unique in that the communication occurs over the telephone as opposed to face-to-face. Non-verbal visual cues become irrelevant as only auditory cues can be picked up and acted upon
  - Introduces self and the role
  - Speaks slowly and clearly
  - Listens patiently
  - Recognizes, acknowledges, and validates staff's concerns and feelings
  - Appropriate non-verbal behaviour, which includes voice pace and tone, eye contact, and facial expression
  - Respects the expertise of the midwife

Information gathering

- Obtains relevant information regarding both patients from the midwife on the telephone

Applied clinical knowledge

- Demonstrates sound and comprehensive evidence-based clinical knowledge and familiarity with the diagnosis and management of puerperal sepsis
- The candidate demonstrates a good knowledge of:
  - Risk factors for puerperal sepsis

- Definition of septic syndromes
- The likely sources of puerperal sepsis
- Microbial profile of the common sources of sepsis of the puerperium
- Antimicrobial use and bacteriological spectrum of activity of common antibiotics
- The clinical features of sepsis, both the symptoms and the signs
- Management of women with sepsis
- Monitoring of women with sepsis
- Red flag signs and symptoms for hospital referral
- Rationale for multi-disciplinary involvement
- Rationale for the investigations
- Infection control issues
- Neo-natal issues
- Surgical considerations.

Notes for Candidate

Multi-disciplinary working is integral to good patient care. This station tests the communication skills of the candidate with allied medical staff as opposed to patients.

This station is also unique in that the communication occurs over the telephone as opposed to face-to-face. Non-verbal visual cues become irrelevant as only auditory cues can be picked up and acted upon. Although this station tests your knowledge, you should not ignore your communications skills in this station.

You are expected to be thoroughly familiar with the RCOG guideline on sepsis.

For the telephone conversation, your questions should cover:

- Introduction over the telephone
- Clinical history
- Risk factors
- Symptoms of sepsis
- Signs of sepsis targeted to identify the source
- Investigations in the Community
- Red flag signs

For the second scenario, concentrate on answering the questions posed by the examiner. Answer to the point.

Further reading

Bacterial Sepsis Following Pregnancy Green-top Guideline No 64b April 2012; RCOG. https://www.rcog.org.uk/globalassets/documents/guidelines/gtg_64b.pdf

Task 5 **Neonatal problems at birth and discussion of these with parents**

Instructions for Candidate

This task assesses the following clinical skills:

- Patient safety
- Communication with patients and their relatives
- Applied clinical knowledge

Mrs. Daniels has delivered a full term baby earlier today. She is with her baby on the postnatal ward.

As a part of the pre-discharge examination of the new born your task is:

- Demonstrate on the anatomical model, the technique for detecting congenital hip dysplasia in the newborn
- Demonstrate the following neonatal reflexes, explaining the expected response in a normal newborn. You will be asked to perform the tasks on a doll. Please treat the doll as a baby:
  - Rooting
  - Walking/Placing
  - Moro/startle reflex
- Explain what conditions are conditions are screened for on the routine newborn blood spot screening test?

You have 10 minutes for this task (+ 2mins initial reading time).

Instructions for Assessor

This clinical assessment task is to assess the candidates' ability to assess a newborn baby's hips and neurological status.

The candidate should examine the model demonstrating the technique used to identify congenital hip dislocation

Then they should perform the following reflexes:

- Rooting
- Walking/Placing
- Moro/startle reflex

Ask them to explain what they are doing while performing the reflex and what would the expected response in a normal newborn be?

Finally, ask the candidate 'Which five conditions are screened for on the routine newborn blood spot screening test?'

Assessment

Marking Scheme

Patient safety:

Pass Borderline Fail

Communication with patients and their relatives:

Pass Borderline Fail

Applied clinical knowledge:

Pass Borderline Fail

Notes for Marking

Patient safety

- Washes hands without a prompt
- Treats the model gently
- Asks permission to examine the neonate
- Clarifies that examination will be performed with the mum present

Communication with patients and their relatives

- Introduces himself/herself to the mother
- Obtains verbal consent
- Explains the process of neonatal reflexes clearly
- Explains the expected response in a newborn clearly

Applied clinical knowledge

- Correctly positions the model
  - Infant supine
  - Legs towards examiner
  - Firm surface
- For Right hip
  - Steadies pelvis with right hand—fingers over sacrum, thumb over pubic symphysis
  - Left hand—finger on great trochanter, thumb in groin over upper femoral shaft
  - Abducts the hip pushing gently backwards with thumb
  - Abducts the hip feeling a definite clunk as the femoral head re-enters the acetabulum
  - Reports that the test is positive/abnormal i.e. dislocated hip
- For left hip—same as described with change of hands

Reflexes

Rooting

Gently stroke the baby on either cheek
Baby turns head on the side of the cheek touched to find breast

Walking/Placing

Hold baby in an upright position, with your hands under their armpits, gently place one of their feet to touch couch.

As feet touch the ground, baby makes walking/stepping motion.

Moro/Startle

Hold supine infant by supporting shoulders/upper back with one hand and support head with other hand. Allow head to drop a short distance into the hand,
gently drop baby back to elicit startle.

Baby throws arms out in extension followed by flexion.

The five conditions screened on routine newborn blood spot test are:

1. Phenylketonuria
2. Congenital hypothyroidism
3. Cystic fibrosis
4. Sickle cell disease
5. MCAD (Medium-chain acyl-CoA Dehydrogenase Deficiency) accept abbreviation

Notes for Candidate

Familiarize yourself with the newborn assessment.

You may wish to shadow your paediatric colleagues, if they do the routine neonatal assessment, in your place of work.

Further reading

StratOG: Examination of the Newborn. https://stratog.rcog.org.uk/tutorial/assessment-of-the-newborn-and-common-neonatal-problems/examination-of-the-newborn-2753

Newborn blood spot test. http://www.nhs.uk/conditions/pregnancy-and-baby/pages/newborn-blood-spot-test.aspx

Task 6 **Ventouse delivery**

Instructions for Candidate

This task assesses the following clinical skills:

- Patient safety
- Communication with patients and their relatives
- Information gathering
- Applied clinical knowledge

You are reviewing the patients on the postnatal ward.

The midwife requests you to speak to a mother who had a ventouse delivery around 18 hrs ago. The ventouse delivery was for prolonged second stage. A metal cup was used. The operative notes state that the ventouse cup slipped, but as there was obvious descent with the ventouse, it was reapplied.

The paediatric doctors had assessed the baby at birth and on this morning's ward round. However, the mum has some questions. She was told the lump on the baby's head before delivery called a caput and another called as chignon that had developed due to the ventouse delivery. She wants to know more about it. She also feels that there is a new lump that had developed on the baby's head. She feels the baby appears a bit sallow.

When you examine the baby, indeed the baby has a large chignon with abrasions around the edges.

There is also a boggy fluctuant lump over the occiput. The swelling is obscuring the posterior fontanelle and crosses the suture lines.

Your task is to:

- Explain what all these different swellings on the baby's head mean
- Explain what the other lump could be
- Organize the next steps of management for the baby
- Answer any questions the mother may have

You have 10 minutes for this task (+ 2mins initial reading time).

Instructions for Assessor

This clinical assessment task assesses the communication skills and application of knowledge regarding foetal skull swellings and trauma associated with operative vaginal delivery.

Please do not interrupt or prompt the candidate. Record your overall clinical impression (Pass/Borderline/Fail) of the Candidate for each of the domain.

Instructions for Role Player

You are Abigail Leadsome, a 38-year-old civil servant. You delivered your first baby, Jonathan, about 18 hrs ago. You had an uncomplicated pregnancy.

You went into spontaneous labour and progressed well until full dilatation.

You had epidural analgesia on board during the labour.

There were no concerns about your baby's health throughout the labour.

You were fully dilated for a good two hours before you had any urge to push.

Once you had the urge, you pushed to the best of your ability, as instructed by the midwife for another hour and a half at least.

The midwife then asked the doctor to assess you. As the delivery was not imminent and the baby did not seem to be in the right position, the doctor explained to you that you will need to undergo what is called as trial of an instrumental delivery.

He explained that the baby was in what is called as a right occipito transverse position and that it had descended beyond what they call station 0, so it was safe to try an instrumental delivery, but as when he examined you during a contraction, there was no further descend, he thought it would be best to deliver you in the theatre where they could proceed to a caesarean section if the instrumental delivery fails. You vaguely remember him telling you that already there was some swelling on the baby's head due to the delay in delivery since full dilatation.

He explained to you that he was going to put a suction cup.

You were then taken to theatre where the doctor applied the suction cup on the baby and you pushed when the midwife asked you to push. He said the baby was coming and then there was a sound as though the suction had come off and indeed it had. The doctor reapplied the suction and Jonathan was born almost 5 hrs since full dilatation.

He had a cup shaped swelling on his head.

Ideas: You wonder if all these swellings and abrasions on little Jonathan could have been avoided if you were allowed to have a vaginal delivery. At the time, you were exhausted and were grateful for the help, but in hindsight you are not sure.

You were told that the baby already had some swelling before delivery, what swelling was that?

Concerns: You are concerned that the cup shaped swelling is still present and the scalp of your baby appears bruised.

You are now all the more concerned as a new boggy swelling has developed. Jonathan does not seem to be settling and his colour appears pale and yellow.

Expectations: You expect the doctor to explain about the swelling in the scalp.

You now know it is called 'chignon'?

Why are there abrasions around the chignon?

When will it go? Do we need to do anything about it?

What is this new swelling?

When the doctor tells you about the investigations that need to be done, you have further questions:

Where exactly is bleeding?

Why did it happen?

What happens next?

Assessment

Marking Scheme

Patient safety:

Pass Borderline Fail

Communication with patients and their relatives:

Pass Borderline Fail

Information gathering:

Pass Borderline Fail

Applied clinical knowledge:

Pass Borderline Fail

Notes for Marking

Patient safety

- Assesses the patient's main concerns and idea
- Explains clearly the different swelling terminologies using diagrams if necessary
- Should be aware that subaponeurotic bleed has the potential to cause a haemorrhagic shock and can be fatal
- Should be aware of the possibility of other head trauma
- Calls for help from the paediatric doctor
- Honest about the incidence of subgaleal haemorrhage being higher with repeated ventouse applications
- A good candidate will indicate that an incident form will be filled up and the case discussed at the governance meeting

Communication with patients and their relatives

- Greets, introduces self and role, checks name
- Consent to proceed and explains nature of interview
- Assesses informant's starting point (what they want to know) and sets the agenda

Providing the explanation

- Tailors information carefully to needs of the patient
- Clear organized explanation in logical sequence
- Chunks: i.e. provides information in reasonable chunks
- Checks understanding. Full marks if does this more than once and gets patient to repeat in their own words
- Screens appropriately *(Is there anything else..?)*
- Language (easily understood, avoids or explains jargon)
- Uses visual aids appropriately e.g. diagrams or uses analogies to aid explanation

Information gathering

- Obtains relevant obstetric history, including the events during delivery and postpartum
- Obtains patient's views, expectations, and concerns regarding her baby

Applied clinical knowledge

- **Caput succedaneum** is a serosanguinous, subcutaneous, extraperiosteal fluid collection with poorly defined margins. It is caused by the pressure of the presenting part against the dilating cervix. It settles in a few days and does not need any treatment
- **Chignon** occurs when, during the creation of a vacuum, the foetal scalp is drawn into the ventouse cup producing the mound of scalp tissue and oedema, the chignon. This usually settles in a few days. It does not need any treatment. There can be bruising and sometimes abrasions due to the ventouse cup especially the metal cup and these do settle down within a few days
- **Subaponeurotic/Sungaleal haemorrhage** is bleeding in the potential space between the periosteum and the scalp galea aponeurosis. Majority of the cases result from repeated ventouse attempts applied to the head at delivery

- **Neonates with subaponeurotic haemorrhage** may develop haemorrhagic shock; therefore the paediatric team will need to be involved urgently
    - The baby will also need its haematocrit value checked
    - It has a high frequency of occurrence of associated head trauma (40%), such as intracranial haemorrhage or skull fracture, therefore further investigations like X-ray or CT will be needed

Prolonged second stage

- For a nulliparous woman:
    - Birth would be expected to take place within three hours of the start of the active second stage in most women
    - Diagnose delay in the active second stage when it has lasted two hours and refer the woman to a healthcare professional trained to undertake an operative vaginal birth if birth is not imminent
    - Risks of both maternal and perinatal adverse outcomes rise with increased duration of the second stage, particularly for duration longer than three hours in nulliparous women and longer than two hours in multiparous women

Further reading

Allen VM, Baskett TF, O'Connell CM, McKeen D, Allen AC. Maternal and perinatal outcomes with increasing duration of the second stage of labor. *Obstetrics & Gynecology*. 2009. 113(6): 1248–58. doi: 10.1097/AOG.0b013e3181a722d6.

StratOG:Forceps and ventouse. https://stratog.rcog.org.uk/tutorial/forceps-and-ventouse/neonatal-injury-2457

Newborn assessment. https://stratog.rcog.org.uk/tutorial/assessment-of-the-newborn-and-common-neonatal-problems/birth-injuries-2783

Nice: Intrapartum care. https://www.nice.org.uk/guidance/cg190

Chapter 14 **Gynaecological problems**

Task 1 **Menstrual disorders**

Instructions for Candidate

This task assesses the following clinical skills:

- Patient safety
- Communication with patients and their relatives
- Information gathering
- Applied clinical knowledge

You are in the gynaecology clinic and your next patient is Rachel Sawyer a 38-year-old woman suffering from heavy and irregular periods. She has a BMI of 42 and has been diagnosed with PCOS in the past.

Your task is

- To take a focussed history
- Explain what examination and investigations need to be performed to Rachel
- Make a management plan

You have 10 minutes for this task (+ 2mins initial reading time).

Instruction for Assessors

Please read instructions to candidate and actor.

Allow the candidate to conduct the interview undisturbed unless they are straying off the track of the question (in which case you can show them their instructions again).

This patient has heavy and irregular periods. The history of presenting complaint should cover:

- The extent, duration, and inconvenience caused by the bleeding
- Establish the menstrual history from menarche
- Last menstrual period and present menstrual cycle
- Past gynaecological history, including PCOS
- No medical, surgical, family history
- No allergies
- Normal and regular smears
- Nulliparous
- Wants to preserve fertility

Once the candidate has taken a relevant history, they are expected to explain that they will need to perform a speculum examination and bimanual examination to Rachel. They should explain that this is to rule out any obvious abnormality in the vagina/cervix and to assess the uterus and adnexa.

Abdominal examination—unremarkable:

- Speculum examination—cervix satisfactory
- Bimanual examination—uterus bulky, retroverted, mobile, no adnexal masses Investigations

- Endometrial sampling—either at this consultation or accept another appointment-This is to assess the endometrium as, although 38, Rachel has risk factors of High BMI, PCOS, and nulliparity
- TVS- as Rachel has a high BMI, the sensitivity of an internal examination is reduced, TVS, not TAS will be useful due to high BMI. Ultrasound to rule out ovarian or uterine pathology as clinically bulky uterus

Management plan

Will depend on the investigations
Addresses weight reduction
Explains the importance of progesterone especially in view of PCOS
Explains the intrauterine system
Record your overall clinical impression of the candidate for each domain (e.g. should this performance be pass, borderline, or a fail)

Instructions for Role Player

You are Rachel Sawyer (38) secretary to a local solicitor. You are suffering from heavy and irregular periods.

You had your first period at age of 12. The periods were initially irregular but not too heavy. At the ago of 14 you went on minipill for contraception and this helped your periods. You came off the pill at the age of 26, as you and your then partner wanted to try for a baby. You tried for about two years without any success. In the mean time your periods became heavier and very irregular.

You used to bleed for anything from seven–21 days every 21–45 days. Periods were very heavy with clots. Unfortunately, your relationship broke down at the same time. You were referred to the hospital by your GP at that time. You underwent an ultrasound and some hormonal blood tests and were diagnosed to have polycystic ovarian syndrome. If asked, you did have a problem with excess upper lip and chin hair. You were started on the contraceptive pills, which were controlling your periods until about 4 years ago. Your GP has tried to change the pill, but without much success. You therefore stopped the pills and over the last year your bleeding has become very heavy and you bleed for prolonged periods of time as before.

You are aware that you are overweight and believe that you eat healthy, but because of the irregular bleeding find it difficult to exercise. You do not smoke.

You have no other medical history. If asked, you have not been tested for diabetes recently.

Although currently not sexually active, you wish to preserve your fertility.

Your last period was two weeks ago and you are still bleeding. Prior to that you bled continuously for four weeks. You currently bleed for anything from 15–13 days and the interval between the two periods can be three to six weeks. Your periods are interfering with your life to an extent that you are getting depressed and have needed to take time off work.

If you are specifically asked:

- In the past you have never had any major illnesses
- You don't have excessive bleeding from elsewhere (e.g. nose bleeds or when you cut yourself)
- You have not undergone any surgeries
- You do not have any relevant family history
- You are not known to be allergic to any medication
- You have no other symptoms (breathing, chest pain, bowels etc)
- No problems with cervical smears

Temperament: You think you are a calm, level-headed woman who can get on with something once you make up your mind about it.

Ideas: You are expecting the doctors to tell you about your weight again!

You are expecting them to organize an ultrasound. You were not expecting the biopsy from the lining of the womb.

Concerns: You are worried that you may not be able to get pregnant.

Expectations: You want the doctor to explain the following:

- Why are they organising the investigations?
- You expect them to explain what endometrial hyperplasia means
- Why the intrauterine system is necessary?
- What will happen to your fertility?

Assessment

Marking Scheme

Pass Borderline Fail

Communication with patients and their relatives:

Pass Borderline Fail

Information gathering:

Pass Borderline Fail

Applied clinical knowledge:

Pass Borderline Fail

Notes for Marking

Patient safety

- Assesses the patient's main concerns
- Involves patient in the process (e.g. encouraging them to express their ideas, or preferences
- Aware of the risk factors for endometrial hyperplasia and ca.
- Negotiates a mutually agreed acceptable, safe, plan
- Open and honest about weight management without being patronising
- Open and honest about the risk of endometrial pathology

Communication with patients and their relatives

- Greets, introduces self and role, checks patient's name
- Consent to proceed and explains nature of interview
- Assesses patient's starting point (what the patient wants to know) and sets the agenda
- Clear organized explanation in logical sequence
- Chunks: e.g. provides information in reasonable chunks
- Checks patient's understanding.
- Language (easily understood, avoids or explains jargon)
- Uses visual aids appropriately e.g. diagrams or uses analogies to aid explanation
- Presents a clear and succinct history to the assessor

Information gathering

- Obtains a relevant gynaecological history
- Obtains patient's views, expectations, and concerns

Applied clinical knowledge

- Demonstrates a sound and comprehensive evidence-based clinical knowledge
- Understands the significance of focussed menstrual history

Notes for Candidate

The scenario is taken from a common clinical scenario of our daily practice. It not only assesses the process of communication but also assesses the content of the knowledge given to the patient. It is important *how* you provide the information to the patient.

Practice this scenario with one of your friends who can act as a role player and ask another friend to provide you with feedback.

Further reading

Heavy menstrual bleeding: assessment and management Clinical guideline [CG44] Published January 2207 Last updated: August 2016. https://www.nice.org.uk/guidance/cg44?unlid=7374295120162942910

Task 2 **Endometriosis**

Instructions for Candidate

This task assesses the following clinical skills:

- Patient safety
- Communication with patients and their relatives
- Information gathering
- Applied clinical knowledge

Amy Lonsdale is a 35-year-old woman who has been referred to the gynaecology clinic with symptoms of pelvic pain and dysmenorrhoea.

Your task is to:

- Obtain a detailed history
- Explain diagnosis to Ms. Lonsdale
- Discuss and agree a management plan with Ms. Lonsdale

Examination findings will be provided on enquiry.

You have 10 minutes for this task (+ 2mins initial reading time).

Instruction for Assessors

This clinical assessment task assesses the candidate's ability to take a focussed gynaecological history and make a management plan based on the results of the ultrasound and laparoscopy for endometriosis.

It should capture all the important aspects of:

- Symptoms—dysmenorrhoea, pelvic pain, and the dyspareunia
- Obstetric history, smear history, and the menstrual history should be elucidated

They should be able to understand the patients concerns and expectations.

When asked regarding examination, only volunteer what is asked:

BMI—28
PA—NAD
PS—NAD
VE—Anteverted. Tender, forniceal tenderness, with fullness in left fornix

Based on these findings, the candidate should organize imaging.

Explain to the patient that the most likely diagnosis is endometriosis.

Once the candidate has decided to organize imaging, please provide them with the ultrasound report (Box 14.1).

They should explain what endometriosis is.

Based on the ultrasound report (endometrioma) they should counsel the patient for a laparoscopy and ovarian cystectomy.

They may wish to refer the patient to an endometriosis centre.

Box 14.1 Ultrasound report

Date: **xx/xx/xxxx**
Name: Amy Lonsdale
Date of Birth: dd/mm/yy

Hospital no: xyx

LMP: 2 weeks ago
History; painful periods, pelvic pain, dyspareunia

Findings:
Normal size anteverted uterus with AP diameter measuring 4cm. Endometrium appears homogenous measuring 11mm. Right ovary normal with few follicles.
Left ovary is enlarged with a cyst measuring 6 cm. It shows homogenous echoes suggestive of endometrioma.
Small amount of free fluid in the pouch of Douglas.
Performed by: xyz

If they have not asked for the ultrasound report, do not volunteer.

Tell them that Amy has now undergone a laparoscopy and show them the first picture of the laparoscopy of the laparoscopy (see Fig. 14.1).

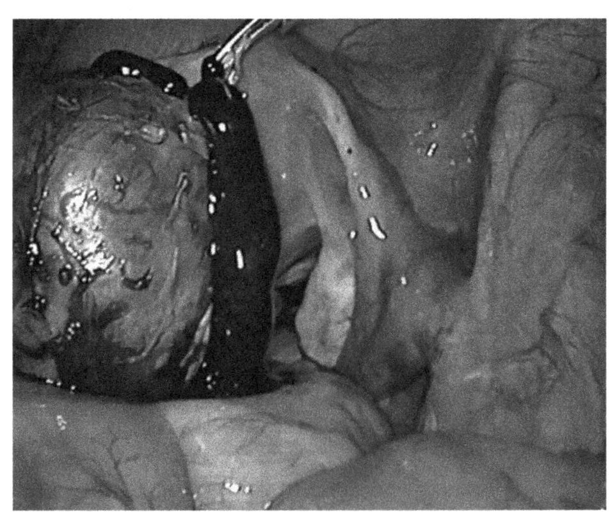

Fig. 14.1 Laparoscopy image

Ask them to comment.

Ask them what would be the right treatment for the endometrioma? (Ovarian cystectomy).

Show them Fig. 14.2 and ask them to comment.

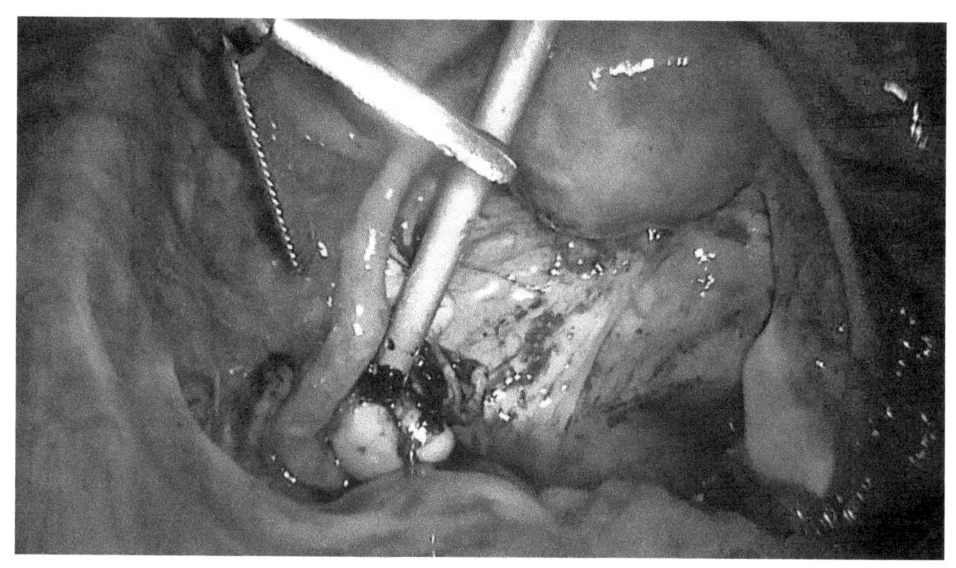

Fig. 14.2 Laparoscopy image

What should be the treatment of the peritoneal endometriosis? (Excision).

Candidates should be able to counsel regarding the implications of endometriosis on infertility. As the patient has undergone endometrioma excision in the form of cystectomy and surgical resection of the endometriosis, this should help with the pain and therefore dyspareunia.

However, fertility does start dropping with age and rapidly after 38, so you would encourage the patient to try and conceive now as it is in her plans already.

If after trying for two years she is unable to conceive, a referral to fertility services should be sought.

As pelvic surgery has been performed, candidates should inform the patient to report early for a scan once pregnant to rule out ectopic pregnancy.

Record your overall clinical impression of the candidate for each domain (i.e. should this performance be pass, borderline, or a fail).

Instructions for Role Player

You are Amy Lonsdale, a local solicitor. You are 35 years of age. You have never been pregnant.

You have always had painful periods. But they have been managed with oral contraceptive pills. But recently, the pain during periods has become excruciating, needing you to take time off work. You have pain all throughout the cycle, but becomes worse midcycle and then around three days prior to your period. It persists throughout the period and then goes back to a dull ache background pain.

Over the last six months you have also been suffering from pain during intercourse, which is deep inside you and again is excruciating.

Your periods had been regular when you were on the contraceptive pills.

You have been in a stable relationship and are now contemplating starting a family and have stopped the pills about six months ago. Since then, your periods are irregular, heavy and you bleed in between periods. Your last period was 1 week ago.

Your pain has become worse.
Your cervical smears have always been normal and regular.
You do not have any major medical or surgical problems.
You are allergic to Penicillin—you had developed an anaphylactic reaction as a child.
You have no relevant family history.

Temperament: You are calm and collected and a professional individual. You like to know your options in detail before contemplating any treatment.

When told that you are likely to have endometriosis, if not volunteered by the candidate, ask:
What is endometriosis?
How do you get it?
When told about laparoscopy and ovarian cystectomy for the endometrioma-ask if not volunteered, how a laparoscopy will be done and the possible complications

Ideas: You are fed up of the pain and really need to get an answer and solution to your problem.

Concerns: You are concerned that as you have left having a child for this long, if there is any problem in your womb or ovaries, this will jeopardize your chances of having a child in the future.
You want to know the implications of the endometrioma on fertility.

Expectations: You are expecting an answer and a plan for your problem. If counselled re medical management, you choose to undergo surgical treatment.

Assessment

Marking Scheme

Pass Borderline Fail

Communication with patients and their relatives:
Pass Borderline Fail

Information gathering:
Pass Borderline Fail

Applied clinical knowledge:
Pass Borderline Fail

Notes for Marking

Patient safety

- Counsels about complications of laparoscopy
- Makes the necessary referrals
- Reads the patients details on the scan report and the ultrasound images Assesses the patient's main concerns and ideas
- Gives options and discusses the pros and cons
- Involves patient in the process (e.g. encouraging them to express their ideas, or preferences)
- Negotiates a mutually agreed acceptable, safe, plan
- Honest—says will seek senior input when does not know the answer

Communication with patients and their relatives

- Greets, introduces self and role, checks patient's name
- Assesses patient's starting point (what the patient wants to know) and sets the agenda
- Clear organized explanation in logical sequence
- Chunks: i.e. provides information in reasonable chunks
- Checks patient's understanding
- Language (easily understood, avoids or explains jargon)
- Uses visual aids appropriately e.g. diagrams or uses analogies to aid explanation

Information gathering

- Obtains a relevant gynaecological history
- Obtains patient's views, expectations, and concerns

Applied clinical knowledge

- History taking—should be aware of the specific symptoms to ask, including dyspareunia
- Should be able to understand the examination findings and organise the necessary investigations—ultrasound
- Will not be wise to undertake laparoscopy without imaging
- Should be aware that ovarian cystectomy is the preferred surgical option to endometrioma drainage and cauterization
- Should be aware that for the extensive peritoneal endometriosis, excision not diathermy should be performed to alleviate patient's symptoms
- Aware of laparoscopy and complications
- Aware of implications of endometriosis, pelvic surgery on fertility

Further reading

Endometriosis, patient information, RCOG, 2007. https://www.rcog.org.uk/globalassets/documents/patients/patient-information-leaflets/gynaecology/endometriosis.pdf

Guideline on Management of Women with endometriosis, ESHRE, 2013. https://www.eshre.eu/Guidelines-and-Legal/Guidelines/Endometriosis-guideline/Guideline-on-the-management-of-women-with-endometriosis.aspx

Task 3 **Paediatric**

Instructions for Candidate

This task assesses the following clinical skills:

- Patient safety
- Communication with patients and their relatives
- Information gathering
- Applied clinical knowledge

You are an ST-5 Doctor working in a gynaecology clinic with your consultant. Your Consultant has asked you to see Miss Julie Smith, a 15-year-old girl who has been referred for 'large labia'. Your task is to:

- Take a detailed history
- Obtain consent for the examination

When these tasks are completed, request the assessor to give you the examination findings. You do not need to examine the patient; however, you do need to explain the process of the examination to the patient. You will be given the examination findings by the assessor.

The proposed management is patient education; no surgical treatment is required. Explain this to the patient and her family and answer their questions.

You have 10 minutes for this task (+ 2mins initial reading time). You can split this up into a five minutes pre-examination and five minutes post-examination consultation.

Instruction for Assessors

Please read the instructions to the candidate and the role player.

Allow the candidate to conduct the interview undisturbed unless they are straying off the track of the question, in which case you show them their instructions again.

Aim to complete the assessment and the history taking in about six minutes to allow six minutes for the candidate to explain the management to the patient. The history should cover all the points mentioned in the mark sheet.

When the candidate has obtained consent for the examination, tell the candidate the examination findings: the labia and the rest of the vulva are entirely normal. Therefore, the plan is patient education and that no surgical management is necessary.

Now ask the candidate to explain and justify this to the patient.

There are two marks for the actress to assign at the end of this station.

Record your overall clinical impression (Pass/Borderline/Fail) of the candidate for each of the four domains.

Instructions for Role Player

You are Miss Julie Smith, aged 15. You are doing well in Year 10 at school, taking eight subjects for GCSE. You had first noticed 'large labia' about one year ago as you do have a tendency to study your body parts now and then.

You then looked at images on the internet and became convinced that your labia are abnormal. You have not discussed this with friends as you found this embarrassing. Over the last few months you have become increasingly self-conscious, such that you have stopped attending swimming classes for fear of unpleasant remarks. You eventually disclosed your concerns to your mum as you feel this problem needs 'sorting out' now, but you do not permit your mum to 'see you'.

You do not have any other concerns with any other body parts. You are not sexually active as you feel that your sexual contact may frown upon this abnormality. You live with your mum (your parents are separated) and younger brother. You have a trusting relationship with your mother.

You had your first period aged 13 and you are now regularly using tampons during your periods. You have no problems with your periods. You are otherwise fit and healthy. You do not take any long term medication, nor have you had any previous surgeries.

Ideas: You believe that your labia are large and that most women have normal labia. You also believe that a 'small operation' can 'sort this out'.

Concerns: You are concerned that these 'abnormal labia' will make you 'stand out' and 'not fit in'. You are concerned about the risks of the operation.

Expectations: You are expecting a local examination. You are expecting the doctor to validate your concerns and agree with you that your labia are abnormal. You are expecting the doctor to agree to an operation. When the doctor does not agree you are shocked initially, but accept that you need to give it more serious consideration. You accept a psychological referral if offered.

Assessment

Marking Scheme

Pass Borderline Fail

Communication with patients and their relatives:

Pass Borderline Fail

Information gathering:

Pass Borderline Fail

Applied clinical knowledge:

Pass Borderline Fail

Notes for Marking

Patient safety

- Assesses the patient's main concern
- Involves the patient and the family in the decision making process
- Improves the patient safety by not confusing consumer satisfaction with clinical effectiveness
- Sensitively enquires about sexual activity and sexual abuse
- Enquires about the views of friends, family, and social media
- Negotiates a mutually agreed plan
- Open and honest about the findings, even when realizing these are at variance with the patient perception
- Open and honest about the treatment, even when realising this may not satisfy the patient

Communication with patients and their relatives

- Greets the patient
- Introduces self and the role

- Confirms patient's and mother's identity
- Explains the nature of the consultation
- Puts the patient at ease
- Speaks slowly and clearly
- Picks and responds to patient's non-verbal cues
- Recognizes, acknowledges and validates patient's concerns and feelings
- Appropriate non-verbal behaviour, which includes voice pace and tone, eye contact, and facial expression
- Acknowledges the disappointment of the patient
- Signposts the patient to the relevant website
- Checks patient's understanding
- Allows patient time to react

Information gathering

- Explores the presenting complaint in detail—the duration of the concern and the impact on everyday life. Further, what exactly is the concern? Is it the feeling of being abnormal or the effect on everyday activities?
- Ensures that the child is the one complaining and not anyone else (Munchausen's by proxy)
- Takes a full history, including past medical and past social history, gynaecological history and social history, including issues at school.
- Involves the parent, but focuses on the child

Applied clinical knowledge

- Demonstrates a sound and comprehensive evidence-based clinical knowledge
- Shares factually correct information with the patient
- Sensitively approaches the presenting complaint with the child
- Obtains consent for the examination from both mother and child and makes an effort to see the child alone, but in the presence of the chaperone
- Explains the examination process to the child and its necessity
- Explains to the patient:
  i. the great variation in the normal size and shape of the vagina
  ii. that there is no relationship between the appearance and function of the labia
  iii. the short term complications of labial surgery
  iv. the long term complications viz: neuropathic pain/permanent injury
  v. that physiological changes continue until around 19 years of age
  vi. the inadvizability of surgery
  vii. Female genital cosmetic surgery is not available on the NHS
- Offers consultant input and psychological support to the patient
- Uses patient information leaflets where available
- Refers to reliable websites for further information

Notes for Candidate

This scenario is now becoming increasingly common. Ensure that you display sensitivity during the consultation, considering the special needs of this vulnerable paediatric or adolescent group. This station assesses the content of the information provided as well as the process of communication.

Legal principles regarding the age of consent should not be overlooked. For further reading refer to *BritSPAG Position Statement on Labial Reduction Surgery*, published October 2013.

You should be aware of **Fraser competence**, as it is increasingly used in broader health issues for younger people.

A summary of five Fraser criteria are:

- According to the Fraser criteria, contraception can be provided if:
- The young person understands the advice given to her by the health care professional
- The young person cannot be persuaded to inform her parents, or to allow the healthcare professional to inform them
- It is likely that the young person will continue to have sexual intercourse, with or without the use of contraception
- The young person's physical or mental health may suffer as a result of withholding contraceptive advice or treatment
- It is in the best interests of the young person for the clinician to provide contraceptive advice or treatment, or both, without parental consent

Although the Fraser criteria, has been traditionally used for providing contraception to young people, its use has also been extended to broader health issues in young people.

Further reading

BritSPAG Position Statement on Labial Reduction Surgery, published October 2013. https://www.rcog.org.uk/globalassets/documents/news/britspag_labiaplastypositionstatement.pdf

Ethical opinion paper Ethical considerations in relation to female genital cosmetic surgery (FGCS), RCOG, RCOG Ethics committee, October 2013. https://www.rcog.org.uk/globalassets/documents/guidelines/ethics-issues-and-resources/rcog-fgcs-ethical-opinion-paper.pdf

Task 4 **Adolescent gynaecology**

Instructions for Candidate

This task assesses the following clinical skills:

- Patient safety
- Communication with patients and their relatives
- Information gathering
- Applied clinical knowledge

You are in clinic. Take a history and formulate an action plan for this 15-year-old patient who has been referred by her GP with irregular menorrhagia.

You have 10 minutes for this task (+ 2mins initial reading time).

Instruction for Assessors

Please read instructions to candidate, actress and her mother.

Allow candidate to conduct the interview.

Observe the consultation skills and management of interaction between mother and daughter.

The candidate should focus on the girl but should not exclude her mother from the consultation.

Record your overall clinical impression of the candidate for each domain (e.g. pass, borderline, or fail).

Instructions for Role Player

You are 15 years old; menarche was at 13 years preceded by both thelarche (breast development) and pubarche (growth of axillary and pubic hair). Your periods have always been heavy but have got worse recently. They last for up to ten days. Your cycle was regular but is now less so, ranging from 35–60 days. You have put on some weight over the past year. Your skin has always been bad (acne). If asked you report some facial hirsutism, but no headaches, visual disturbance or milky secretion from your breasts.

You are doing all right at school but have been bullied over your weight. You do have a boyfriend but have not had intercourse—although you think you might like to do this (your mother is not aware). If the doctor suggests that you take the COCP then you would welcome this.

Your mother has accompanied you to the clinic. She is concerned that you are sexually active with your boyfriend and would not be keen for you to start the COCP.

Concerns: You are concerned about your increase in weight, your acne and what other people think about you. You are also worried about contraception if you and your boyfriend decide to have sex.

Expectations: You hope that the doctor will explain why your periods have become irregular and heavy and that they will suggest some treatment that will help.

Mother's concerns and expectations: You have been finding your daughter increasingly moody and difficult. You don't like her boyfriend and are worried that if the doctor prescribes the pill she will have sex.

Assessment

Marking Scheme

Pass Borderline Fail

Communication with patients and their relatives:

Pass Borderline Fail

Information gathering:

Pass Borderline Fail

Applied clinical knowledge:

Pass Borderline Fail

Notes for Marking

Patient safety

- Assesses risk of pregnancy
- Makes a diagnosis from history and results of investigations
- Excludes coagulation defects
- Discusses long term risks of PCOS with patient including diabetes and endometrial hyperplasia

Communication with patients and their relatives

- Greets, introduces self and role, and checks names
- Explains what they are going to do
- Places teenager at centre of consultation
- Involves mother in discussion
- Respects confidentiality of teenager (can exclude mother from some parts of conversation)
- Negotiates management plan with girl and explains this to daughter and mother
- Communicating with colleagues
- Presents history to assessor

Information gathering

- Obtains clinical history including patient's concerns and expectations
- Also takes into account mother's concerns

Applied clinical knowledge

- Aware of most likely diagnosis—PCOS—and Rotterdam criteria for making this diagnosis
- Discusses appropriate management including weight loss and ensuring withdrawal bleed at least every three months

- Excludes other causes for symptoms—e.g. coagulation disorders, other reasons for oligomenorrhoea and hyperandrogenism

Notes for Candidate

This scenario tests your ability to manage an adolescent consultation and negotiate a plan for investigation and management.

The adolescent consultation can be challenging—the adolescent may be reluctant to volunteer information and may be embarrassed. It is important to make the adolescent central to the consultation and not allow mother 'to take over'. It is also important to try and separate mother and daughter so that you can ask about sexual activity away from the mother.

The working diagnosis in this case is anovulatory heavy bleeds probably secondary to PCOS that has been 'activated' by weight gain. However, it is also important to explore the possibility of coagulation defects (e.g. easy bruising, epistaxis, family history). The symptoms may also represent 'normal' adolescent menstruation that has not yet settled to an adult pattern.

Therefore investigations are organized to exclude anaemia and a coagulation defect and to assess for PCOS and should include—USS pelvis, FBC +/- coagulation, +/- Von Willebrand factor assessment, day two gonadotrophins and oestradiol, prolactin, thyroid function tests and androgens (testosterone and 17OH progesterone).

If PCOS is confirmed then management involves normalization of weight and either one week courses of Norethisterone to induce a withdrawal bleed every three months if the patient is having less frequent menstrual bleeds, or the COCP taken cyclically. Selecting a COCP with an anti-androgenic progestogen will help acne and hirsutism (e.g. Dianette). If the COCP is advised this will need careful counselling of daughter and mother given the background.

Abnormal vaginal bleeding after the menarche

Most cycles following the onset of menstruation are anovular and irregular for at least the first two years. Once ovulation is established bleeding patterns will regularize but this can take up to seven years. Young patients (and their doctors) need to understand what is normal so education is an important part of management.

Acute adolescent menorrhagia is associated with a primary coagulation disorder in up to 20% of cases. Von Willebrand's disease is the most common. The haemoglobin level can be used to decide treatment. This can, if the patient is not anaemic, be conservative combined with educating the patient. Alternatively, oral anti fibrinolytics, NSAIDs and the COCP can be used. Cerazette or an IUS are other options but do not address the underlying cause of anovular cycles and low oestrogen, which are better addressed by management of the underlying disorder—in this case PCOS.

Polycystic ovarian syndrome and hyperandrogenism

PCOS is a heterogenous collection of signs and symptoms. The diagnosis is currently made using the Rotterdam criteria. Patients need two out of the three following criteria (chronic anovulation, clinical or biochemical hyperandrogenism and polycystic ovaries on scan) with exclusion of other aetiologies (congenital adrenal hyperplasia, Cushing's syndrome). Management depends on the patient's main concerns. (E.g. hirsutism, infertility, weight gain.) The clinician also needs to be aware of long term complications including diabetes and endometrial hyperplasia and carcinoma.

In this case inducing regular withdrawal bleeds with either the COCP or three monthly courses of progestogens will reduce the risk of developing endometrial hyperplasia. The COCP may reduce clinical hyperandrogenism. Reducing weight however, remains the mainstay of treatment.

Adolescents are rarely concerned with their future fertility—but their mothers may be. It is important that appropriate counselling is given regarding the need for contraception if sexually active, even if the patient is amenorrhoeic.

Notes on adolescent gynaecology

Adolescent gynaecology includes a wide range of conditions in post pubertal females up to age 20 years. The consultation can be challenging; the adolescent should be central to any discussion. Management is often conservative. Doctors need to acquire additional knowledge and skills to provide optimal care. They should be able to recognize unusual conditions including disorders of sexual differentiation and be able to provide counselling and appropriate referral.

The WHO defines adolescence as between ten and 20 years. It is characterized by rapid development in psychological, social and biological domains. Adolescent gynaecology includes a wide range of conditions, many of which may also present in older females. Although conditions may be familiar to gynaecologists more used to adults, the consultation can be challenging and subsequent management, which is often conservative, may differ. Doctors need to acquire additional knowledge and skills in order to provide optimal care. In addition, it is important to be able to recognize unusual conditions and refer appropriately. Common conditions include menstrual dysfunction, dysmenorrhea and pelvic pain, ovarian cysts, polycystic ovarian syndrome (PCOS), hyperandrogenism, and oligo and amenorrhoea. Less common presentations include primary or premature ovarian insufficiency, requests for fertility preservation pre and post oncology treatment, delayed puberty, the female athletic triad and disorders of sexual differentiation.

Key knowledge

1. Understanding of puberty including hormonal changes.
2. Understanding of normal sexual development and differentiation.
3. Understanding social, educational and psychological changes taking place in adolescence.
4. The hypothalamic- pituitary—ovarian axis.
5. The menstrual and ovarian cycles.
6. Aetiology of oligomenorrhoea and amenorrhoea.
7. Consent and confidentiality in adolescents (Gillick competence and Fraser guidelines).

Key skills

1. The consultation with the adolescent +/- her parents. Communication skills specific to adolescent consultation.
2. Appropriate examination—Tanner staging and examination external genitalia.

In Paediatric and Adolescent Gynaecology (PAG) clinical assessment tasks may be used to assess a candidate's ability to manage a consultation, to obtain consent in a patient < 16 years, to provide disclosure of a diagnosis for example the XY female or to differentiate between common and rare conditions which need onward referral (for example intact hymen versus transverse vaginal septae).

Further reading

Garden A, Hernon M, Topping J. *Paediatric & Adolescent Gynaecology for the MRCOG and beyond.* 2nd Edition. 2008. Cambridge: Cambridge University Press.

Balen A, Creighton SC, Davies M, MacDougall J & Stanhope R, eds. *Mulitidisciplinary approach to the Management of Paediatric & Adolescent Gynaecology.* (2004) . Cambridge: Cambridge University Press.

MacDougall J. Paediatric & Adolescent problems. in *Oxford Desk Reference Obstetrics & Gynaecology.* Arulkumaran S, Regan L, Papageorghiou AT, Monga A, Farquharson DIM eds. 2011. Pp. 570–3. Oxford: Oxford University Press.

Task 5 **Pelvic Pain**

Instructions for Candidate

This task assesses the following clinical skills:

- Patient safety
- Communication with patients and their relatives
- Information gathering
- Applied clinical knowledge

You are an ST4 doctor working in a gynaecology clinic with your consultant. Your consultant has asked you to take relevant history from Julie Wright who is a 30-year-old secretary.

Your task is to:

- Take a brief history. You do not need to examine her, or make a diagnosis
- Summarize the relevant points in the history to the assessor
- Explain diagnostic laparoscopy to Julie

You will be given the examination findings and asked some questions by the assessor.

You have 10 minutes for this task (+ 2mins initial reading time).

Instruction for Assessors

Please read instruction to candidate and actor.

Allow the candidate to conduct the interview undisturbed unless they are straying off the track of the question (in which case you can show them their instructions again).

This patient has pelvic pain and heavy periods the history of presenting complaint should cover

- the extent, duration and inconvenience caused by the pain and bleeding
- Sexual history e.g. dysparuenia
- intermenstural or post coital bleeding
- previous medical interventions
- smear history
- family planning issues
- other bleeding tendency
- PMH and PSH
- family history, social history and current drug history

Once the candidate has taken a relevant history and *presented* to you, provide the candidate with following information:

- Abdominal examination—unremarkable
- Speculum examination—cervix satisfactory
- Bimanual examination—uterus bulky, retroverted, no adnexal masses but mobility slightly restricted, pouch of Douglas tender
- Trans-abdominal and trans-vaginal scan
- Bladder not full, trans-vaginal scan was carried out with verbal consent
- A-P diameter 5.2cm, endometrial thickness 12mm, the endometrium was clearly visualized. Left ovary appeared normal, right ovary was not visualized. Small amount of free fluid in the pouch of Douglas. The patient found transvaginal scan uncomfortable.

Plan: *For a diagnostic laparoscopy at day procedure unit.*

Now ask the candidate to explain the management plan to Mrs J Wright.

There are some marks on the process mark sheet for the actor to assign at the end of the station.

Record your overall clinical impression of the candidate for each domain (i.e. should this performance be pass, borderline, or a fail).

Instructions for Role Player

You are Julie Wright, aged 30. You are married to John who works as a cleaner in the council offices. You have a five-year-old son, Sam from your previous relationship. You plan to have one more child from your current relationship but are not yet considering getting pregnant. You work part time as a secretary but recently have been off sick on several occasions for lower abdominal pain. An ultrasound scan arranged by your doctor was reported normal. Your doctor treated you with some antibiotics and painkillers. However, you have not noticed any difference to your pain. As you have not responded to treatment you and your gynaecologist have agreed that a laparoscopy (looking inside your tummy with a telescope) is the next step.

You have always had quite painful periods but in the last two to three years since you met John they have become increasingly painful, particularly a week before the onset of your periods. Sexual intercourse is increasingly becoming painful and has reached a point that you do not look forward to it anymore. You have had to take quite a few days off work because of pain and bleeding and encountered embarrassing accidents on several occasions. You bleed for around seven to ten days and for the first four you always have clots and need to use towels as well as tampons every few hours. You need to wake at least a couple of times at night to change or you will stain the bedclothes. You do not have any bleeding in between your periods or after intercourse.

If you are specifically asked:

- In the past you have never had any major illnesses and apart from having your impacted wisdom teeth out under general anaesthetic (which went fine) you haven't had an operation before• You don't have excessive bleeding from elsewhere (e.g. nose bleeds or when you cut yourself)
- You are taking tranexamic acid (which is supposed to help the bleeding but never seem to make any difference) and no other pills (you use the condom for contraception)
- You were adopted and have no idea about family history
- You have no other symptoms (breathing, chest pain, bowels etc)
- No problems with cervical smears

Temperament: You think you are a calm, level headed woman who can get on with something once you make up your mind about it.

Ideas: You were expecting that an ultrasound scan will be necessary and will provide you with the answer to the cause of your pain. You were not expecting any operation.

Concerns: You are worried that you may have some abnormality inside your tummy, which may prevent you to get pregnant.

You are scared to have an operation, and want to find out more about laparoscopy.

Expectations: You want the doctor to explain the following:

- Alternative to laparoscopy
- The procedure itself
- Risks and benefits associated with the procedure
- Who will be doing it?
- What happens if there are complications? What is the chance of anything going wrong during your operation?

- Can anything be done to reduce the chance of having any complication?
- When can you go back to work?

Assessment

Marking Scheme

Pass Borderline Fail

Communication with patients and their relatives:

Pass Borderline Fail

Information gathering:

Pass Borderline Fail

Applied clinical knowledge:

Pass Borderline Fail

Notes for Marking

Patient safety

- Assesses the patient's main concerns and ideas
- Gives options and discusses the pros and cons of laparoscopy
- Discusses possible complications and measures to reduce them
- Involves patient in the process (e.g. encouraging them to express their ideas, or preferences)
- Negotiates a mutually agreed acceptable, safe, plan
- Open and honest about procedure and possible complications
- Provides with information about the person performing the procedure and safeguard in place i.e. competent clinician or junior doctor under direct supervision
- Explain mechanism in place to deal with complications and learn from such complications
- Being honest about prolongation of recovery time if untoward complication happen

Communication with patients and their relatives

- Greets, introduces self and role, checks patient's name
- Consent to proceed and explains nature of interview
- Assesses patient's starting point (what the patient wants to know) and sets the agenda
- Clear organized explanation in logical sequence
- Chunks: i.e. provides information in reasonable chunks
- Checks patient's understanding.
- Language (easily understood, avoids or explains jargon)
- Uses visual aids appropriately e.g. diagrams or uses analogies to aid explanation
- Presents a clear and succinct history to the assessor

Information gathering

- Obtains a relevant gynaecological history
- Obtains patient's views, expectations, and concerns

Applied clinical knowledge

- Demonstrates a sound and comprehensive evidence-based clinical knowledge—i.e. confirms standard practice and reiterates laparoscopy as gold standard test for pelvic pain
- Counsels the patient with relevant information that is factually correct.- pelvic tenderness, dyspareunia Tender POD pointing towards a diagnosis of possible endometriosis
- Discusses alternative management plan i.e. medical treatment with GnRh analogues
- Justify management plan

Notes for Candidates

The scenario is taken from a common clinical scenario of our daily practice. It not only assesses the process of communication but also assesses the content of the knowledge given to the patient. Important thing is how you provide the information to the patient. Practice this scenario with one of your friends who can act as a role player and ask another friend to provide you the feedback.

Further reading

Diagnostic laparoscopy, Consent advice No.2, RCOG, 2008. https://www.rcog.org.uk/globalassets/documents/guidelines/ca2-15072010.pdf

Task 6 **Pelvic pain**

Instructions for Candidate

This task assesses the following clinical skills:

- Patient safety
- Communication with patients and their relatives
- Information gathering
- Applied clinical knowledge

You are in the gynaecology clinic and have been asked to see Sophie Harmer.

She is a 33-year-old lady who has been amenorrhoeic for nine months and wishes to have another child.

She has had normal cervical smears, is in otherwise in good health with no significant medical history and no previous surgery except for delivery of a baby boy by caesarean section four years ago. There is no family history of early menopause. Her mother's menopause was about 48 years of age.

She neither smokes nor drinks alcohol, and has a body mass index of 25. Examination is otherwise normal.

Her GP requested a pelvic ultrasound scan and serum hormone profile. Sophie has yet to have these results discussed with her.

Pelvic ultrasound—normal uterus, AP diameter 4.2cm, no focal fibroids, endometrial thickness 3mm. Right ovary small measuring 2.2 x 2.9cm, left ovary not seen due to overlying bowel gas. No free fluid.

Hormone profile:

Thyroid function, FBC liver function and renal function all normal

Serum estradiol 98pmol/l

Serum FSH—48mIU/l

Take a relevant history, explain the implications of the above test results and discuss with the patient her ongoing management

You have 10 minutes for this task (+2mins initial reading time).

Instruction for Assessors

This station is designed to test the student's ability to take a relevant history, break the provisional potentially bad news of a diagnosis of premature ovarian insufficiency in a sympathetic manner and make an appropriate initial plan of management, all underpinned by knowledge of recent NICE guidance in the diagnosis and management of POI.

Note the terms 'premature menopause' and 'premature ovarian failure' are now considered outdated.

Record your overall clinical impression of the candidate for each domain (i.e. should this performance be pass, borderline, or a fail).

Instructions for Role Player

You are Sophie Harmer, a 33-year-old lady who, over the past nine months has been amenorrhoeic. You are not using contraception as you would like to have another baby. You have one child, a boy, delivered by caesarean section due to a long labour four years ago.

You have had normal cervical smears and are otherwise in good health with no significant medical history and no previous surgery except for the caesarean section.

You work as an admin officer for a local large insurance company. You do not smoke, drink no alcohol, and have a body mass index of 25.

You are married to Chris Harmer, a 39-year-old highly successful IT consultant who works long hours. He is fit and healthy but is indifferent to your wish for a second child. Whilst this is not causing conflict in your relationship because you haven't been using contraception for at least two years your outward indifference is hiding a stronger internal desire for a baby. You have always wanted a daughter. You are clear, however, that under no circumstances would either of you want to pursue fertility treatment to conceive. It either happens naturally or not at all.

You went to see your GP about the above and she was very sympathetic but said that you needed to see a gynaecologist. She requested some blood tests and an ultrasound scan. You have not yet had these results explained to you and one of your expectations of this gynaecology clinic appointment is to discuss the results with a gynaecologist.

Your underlying suspicion is that you have gone through an early menopause. You have kept the symptoms hidden from your husband and your GP. You are not sleeping due to night sweats and you are not coping well at work and your husband's long hours are not helping with the juggling.

The candidate is likely to ask you about your main concerns—try to be brief. On one hand you are devastated that this first test suggests that you have had a premature menopause. Outward emotion (whatever seems most appropriate) could be relief that you have confirmation of a diagnosis. It could be tears about the daughter you won't have or it could be optimism because something could be done to help you feel better than you do now.

Be prepared to get emotional or even cross if the candidate doesn't break the news sympathetically. Ask about HRT. You've heard it has risks. Be easily reassured if the candidate is appropriately clear in his/her reassurance. Be happy to take HRT. If they start talking about contraception just say you don't need it and would be happy if you were to conceive.

You should also have another blood test within six weeks of the first. If not already raised by the candidate, ask them for follow-up plans or ask them if they are certain about the diagnosis.

Assessment

Marking Scheme

Pass Borderline Fail

Communication with patients and their relatives:

Pass Borderline Fail

Information gathering:

Pass Borderline Fail

Applied clinical knowledge:

Pass Borderline Fail

Notes for Marking

Patient safety

- Assesses the patient's main concerns
- Involves patient in the process (e.g. encouraging them to express their ideas, or preferences)

- Negotiates a mutually agreed acceptable, safe, plan to include use of hormone replacement and follow-up until stable symptomatically
- Open and honest about the situation without being patronising
- Open and honest about the long term implications of POI
- Offer to help explain diagnosis to husband if she wishes

Communication with patients and their relatives

- Greets patient and obtains patient's name
- Introduces self, role
- Ability to take a short, relevant history
- Explains nature of interview (reason for coming to talk to patient)
- Assesses starting point: ideas, concerns, and expectations
- Breaks the bad news in an appropriate fashion.
- Use of the 'warning shot' and attentive listening
- Gives clear signposting
- Chunks and checks, using patient's response to guide next steps
- Gives explanation in an organized manner (signposting/summarising)
- Uses clear language, avoids jargon and confusing language
- Picks up and responds to patient's non-verbal cues
- Recognizes, acknowledges and validates patient's concerns and feelings (e.g. uses empathy)
- Appropriate non-verbal behaviour e.g. eye contact, posture and position, movement, facial expression, use of voice (pace, tone)
- Provides support: e.g. concern, understanding, willingness to help
- Arranges review appointment
- Points towards information sources such as Daisy Network Patient support group in the UK

Information gathering

- Obtains a relevant gynaecological history
- Obtains patient's views, expectations, and concerns

Applied clinical knowledge

- Demonstrates a sound and comprehensive evidence-based clinical knowledge of the diagnosis and management of POI
- Is aware that her previous history could have a bearing on the aetiology but there are no clear signs of this
- A diagnosis of POI would be based on:
  - Symptoms experienced—in this case amenorrhoea and night sweats
  - And raised FSH levels on two occasions four to six weeks apart
- POI should not be diagnosed after one blood test
- Routine use of anti-Müllerian hormone levels should not be performed to diagnose POI
- If in doubt consider referral to a specialist menopause clinic
- Either the combined oral contraceptive pill or systemic HRT are considered appropriate treatments at the moment, coming down to patient choice. RCTs have not yet established superiority of one treatment over another

- Warn may still conceive so needs to consider contraceptive needs
- Long term risks—osteoporosis, cardiovascular disease, urogenital implications

Further reading

Menopause: diagnosis and management, NICE guideline [ng23] Published date: November 2015. https://www.nice.org.uk/guidance/ng23/ifp/chapter/About-this-information

Task 7 **Menopause**

Instructions for candidate

This task assesses the following clinical skills:

- Patient safety
- Communication with patients and their relatives
- Information gathering
- Applied clinical knowledge

You are in the gynaecology clinic and have been asked to see Constance Williams

She is a 53-year-old woman who has been amenorrhoeic for six months with severe hot flushes and debilitating night sweats with vaginal dryness and dyspareunia.

She has had normal cervical smears, is in otherwise in good health with no significant medical history and no previous surgery and two term vaginal deliveries in her 20s.

She smokes five to ten cigarettes per day, drinks no alcohol and has a body mass index of 39. Examination is otherwise normal.

She wishes to explore HRT as a possible treatment for her problems.

Take a relevant history and discuss with the patient the benefits and risks of appropriate management strategies.

You have 10 minutes for this task (+ 2mins initial reading time).

Instruction for Assessors

This station is designed to test the student's ability to take a relevant history, explore a patient's background and understanding of menopause, simple lifestyle changes, risks with obesity and in particular Breast cancer risk with HRT.

Record your overall clinical impression of the candidate for each domain (i.e. should this performance be pass, borderline, or a fail).

Instructions for Role Player

You are Constance Williams, a 53-year-old lady who, over the past six months has been amenorrhoeic and has had increasing symptoms of poor performance at work with episodic hot flushes. You are experiencing debilitating night sweats to the point that you wake up in a pool of sweat two to three times per night. Your concentration and short term memory are poor.

You also complain of vaginal dryness and painful sex. These symptoms, in combination with your hot flushes have resulted in a loss of libido, even though you have a strong and loving relationship. Please do not divulge this section of history if the candidate does not put you at ease.

You have had normal cervical smears and one mammogram so far which was normal. You are otherwise in good health with no significant medical history and no previous surgery. You had two term vaginal deliveries in your 20s.

You work as a sales manager in a clothes department in a retail store and your colleagues have noticed your hot flushes and sweats which you find embarrassing. You smoke five to ten cigarettes per day, drink no alcohol and are overweight with a body mass index of 39.

You have tried some natural therapies so far these did not work well, have read about Hormone Replacement Therapy and are pretty convinced you would like to take it.

Before doing so you wish to understand what the main risks of HRT are and whether there are any ways of mitigating these.

The candidate is likely to ask you about your main concerns—try to be brief. Show obvious embarrassment about the effects at work and on your sex life. You are concerned that a work you could lose your job and whilst you and your husband are still very much in love you find talking about sex very embarrassing and you worry about possible long term relationship effects.

You are quite prepared to accept the various risks shown to you as long as they are clear, make sense and are well explained. For all the risks it is reasonable for them to say very small except for breast cancer where you are particularly keen to get a number ('is there a percent increase doc?'). If the candidate goes straight into an explanation of HRT without talking about things you can do yourself (exercise, lose weight, stop smoking, balanced diet) then you should not let those go.

If not covered ask specifically about how you can improve your sex life.

Assessment

Marking Scheme

Pass   Borderline   Fail

Communication with patients and their relatives:

Pass   Borderline   Fail

Information gathering:

Pass   Borderline   Fail

Applied clinical knowledge:

Pass   Borderline   Fail

Notes for Marking

Patient safety

- Assesses the patient's main concerns
- Involves patient in the process (e.g. encouraging them to express their ideas, or preferences)
- Negotiates a mutually agreed acceptable, safe, plan
- Open and honest about the situation without being patronising
- Open and honest about the risks

Communication with patients and their relatives

- Greets patient and obtains patient's name
- Introduces self, role
- Explains nature of interview (reason for coming to talk to patient)
- Assesses starting point: ideas, concerns, and expectations
- Ability to take a short, relevant history
- Places patient at ease, enough to elicit sexual problems
- Gives clear signposting
- Chunks and checks, using patient's response to guide next steps
- Gives explanation in an organized manner (signposting/summarising)
- Uses clear language, avoids jargon and confusing language
- Picks up and responds to patient's non-verbal cues
- Recognizes, acknowledges and validates patient's concerns and feelings (e.g. uses empathy)

- Appropriate non-verbal behaviour e.g. eye contact, posture and position, movement, facial expression, use of voice (pace, tone)
- Provides support: e.g. concern, understanding, willingness to help
- Arranges review appointment
- Points towards information sources

Information gathering

- Obtains a relevant gynaecological history
- Obtains patient's views, expectations, and concerns

Applied clinical knowledge

- Demonstrates a sound and comprehensive evidence-based clinical knowledge of lifestyle measure and benefits/risks of HRT
- Explains ways to reduce hot flushes—weight loss, non-hormonal treatments such as SSRI (but evidence poor for SSRI long term). HRT very effective in over 80%
- Additional benefits of HRT—joint aches, concentration, sleep, work performance
- Longer term benefits—prevention of osteoporosis and possible reduction of risk of CVD if started early in menopause
- Recognizes smoking and obesity along with improving diet main areas to address
- Explains CVD and diabetes significant risks from her obesity and much higher than theoretical risks of HRT
- Less frequent risks—very small increase in absolute risks of stroke and VTE
- Breast cancer and risk—background risk about 23:1000 women aged 50–59 over five years. Four extra cases in combined HRT users, three extra cases in smokers and 24 extra cases in women with BMI >30. Exercise reduces risk
- Discusses hormonal and non-hormonal management of dyspareunia and vaginal dryness. Vaginal moisturisers and lubricants for sex help some. Suggest vaginal oestrogen, licensed for indefinite use with minimal absorption when ten microgram pessaries used twice weekly

Further reading

Menopause: diagnosis and management, NICE guideline [ng23] Published date: November 2015. https://www.nice.org.uk/guidance/ng23/ifp/chapter/About-this-information

Task 8 **Ovarian cysts**

Instructions for Candidate

This task assesses the following clinical skills:

- Patient safety
- Communication with patients and their relatives
- Information gathering
- Applied clinical knowledge

You are the ST5 in the clinic. Your next patient is Rebecca Lee.
Your task is to:

- Take a focused history
- Agree on a management plan
- Counsel her regarding her chosen management option.

You are provided with a GP referral letter (see Box 14.2):
You have 10 minutes for this task (+ 2mins initial reading time).

Instruction for Assessors

This clinical assessment task station assesses the candidate's ability to take a focused history and then discuss the management options in a young lady with a single ovary presented with a persistent ovarian cyst.

It also assesses the candidate's ability to take into consideration the specific circumstances in this case and individualize the plan.

Box 14.2 GP letter

Dear Gynaecologist,
Rebecca is a 27-year-old woman who sadly had a missed miscarriage at ten weeks gestation. At the booking scan three months ago, Rebecca was found to have an unilocular left ovarian cyst measuring 5cms.
I organized a repeat ultrasound, which now shows the presence of the left ovarian cyst measuring 6cms. It has been reported as an unilocular cyst with no suspicious features.
I have attached the ultrasound report.

Thank you
Dr. A. Smith

Ultrasound report
Date: 2 weeks ago
Trans abdominal and transvaginal ultrasound with permission and chaperone
Uterus is anteverted and normal in size and texture. AP diameter is 4.4cms and endometrium (ET) is 0.9cm.
Previous right oophorectomy is noted.
There is a 6cms, unilocular cyst arising from the left ovary.
There are no suspicious features.

Rebecca is asymptomatic therefore conservative management can be considered. However, she needs to be counselled regarding the risks of waiting. Similarly as she has only one ovary and is keen that the cyst is treated, laparoscopic ovarian cystectomy can be offered. Again the candidates should discuss the pros and cons of the procedure.

They should be able to counsel the patient/actor re the options including laparoscopy and discuss the primary open entry (Hassan) and Palmers point entry.

Record your overall clinical impression of the candidate for each domains (i.e. should this performance be pass, borderline, or a fail).

Instructions for Role Player

You are Rebecca Lee. You are a 27-year-old practise nurse at a local GP surgery.

You are generally fit and well.

You do not suffer from any ongoing medical problems.

You have had an operation through an up and down incision starting from your belly button when you were 19. You had a 16cms ovarian cyst on the right ovary. You were rushed in to the hospital with excruciating pain. The doctors told you that the fallopian tube and ovary on the right had to be removed as it had undergone torsion and was dead (necrosed).

You then had an infection of the wound and needed re-suturing of the incision.

You are allergic to Penicillin.

You are adopted and therefore not aware of any family history.

You live with your partner Tom who is a farmer. You both are desperate to start a family.

Temperament: You are generally a calm and collected person. However, you like to know the details. As a health professional you are very much aware of the possible complications and would want to know the risks and benefits in detail.

Ideas: You want the cyst removed and your ovary conserved. You are worried about undergoing another laparotomy and are very keen to have a key hole surgery.

Concerns: You are very upset and concerned.

You were worried after the removal of your right tube and ovary, regarding the implications on your fertility. You were told at the time of surgery that your left tube and ovary are normal.

However, since the detection of the cyst on your left ovary, you have been very worried as you do not want the same problem like last time and then you will be left with no ovaries!

You are also upset as you have undergone a miscarriage recently and you are desperate to start a family.

You are aware of that a previous laparotomy can increase the risk at laparoscopy and want to know how those can be minimized.

Expectations: You expect the doctor to be sympathetic towards your concerns. You expect the doctor to discuss the options, although you want to undergo the key hole surgery to remove the cyst as soon as possible.

You also want to know the implications of all this on your fertility.

You expect the doctor to counsel you regarding how the procedure will be done and the potential risks.

Assessment

Marking Scheme

Pass Borderline Fail

Communication with patients and their relatives:

Pass Borderline Fail

Information gathering:

Pass Borderline Fail

Applied clinical knowledge:

Pass Borderline Fail

Notes for Marking

Patient safety

- Assesses the patient's main concerns and ideas
- Gives options and discusses the pros and cons of each
- Involves patient in the process (e.g. encouraging them to express their ideas, or preferences)
- Negotiates a mutually agreed acceptable, safe, plan
- open and honest
- Honest discussion about the pros and cons of conservative management and surgery

Communication with patients and their relatives

- Greets, introduces self and role, checks patient's name
- Consent to proceed and explains nature of interview
- Assesses patient's starting point (what the patient wants to know) and sets the agenda
- Clear organized explanation in logical sequence
- Chunks: i.e. provides information in reasonable chunks
- Checks patient's understanding.
- Language (easily understood, avoids or explains jargon)
- Uses visual aids appropriately e.g. diagrams or uses analogies to aid explanation

Information gathering

- Obtains a relevant gynaecological history
- Obtains patient's views, expectations, and concerns

Applied clinical knowledge

- A serum CA-125 assay is not necessary when a clear ultrasonographic diagnosis of a simple ovarian cyst has been made

- As the cyst measures 6cms and is noted to be unilocular and the patient is asymptomatic, conservative management with yearly ultrasound follow-up and if the cyst increases to 7cms or larger should be considered for either further imaging (MRI) or surgical intervention
- However, Rebecca should be counselled regarding the cyst accidents, namely rupture and torsion
- Noting that the cyst has not disappeared in more than three months, Rebecca should be counselled that this cyst is unlikely to be physiological
- Surgical option in the form of laparoscopic cystectomy should be discussed
- In view of the previous midline incision, open entry technique or entry through palmers point should be discussed when specifically asked by Rebecca
- The laparoscopic cystectomy should be performed by a suitably qualified surgeon
- Procedure of laparoscopic cystectomy, including the procedure, risks and need for additional procedures including laparotomy and oophorectomy should be discussed
- Repeated pelvic surgery increases the risk of ectopic pregnancy

Further reading

Management of Suspected Ovarian Masses in Premenopausal Women Green–top Guideline No. 62 Joint RCOG/BSGE Guideline I November 2011.

Diagnostic Laparoscopy (Consent Advice No. 2), RCOG. https://www.rcog.org.uk/globalassets/documents/guidelines/ca2-15072010.pdf

Chapter 15 **Subfertility**

Task 1 **Anovulatory infertility**

Instructions for Candidate

This task assesses the following clinical skills:

- Patient safety
- Communication with patients and their relatives
- Information gathering
- Applied clinical knowledge

You are a ST4 doctor working in an infertility clinic. A couple who were referred to the clinic by their GP have returned for review. She has had oligomenorrhoea for the past year. She does not report headaches, visual disturbance, galactorrhoea or hyperandrogenism, she has been trying to conceive for two years. Her partner had an orchidopexy at the age of two.

The assessor will ask you some questions and then give you the results of their investigations. You will be asked to explain the results and next steps to the patient.

You have 10 minutes for this task (+ 2mins initial reading time).

Instructions for Assessor

Please check that candidate and actor have read instructions.

Ask the candidate what investigations they would like to organize for this patient and her partner.

Give them the results of investigations (if asked for):

Pregnancy test—ve

LH 45, FSH 40, E2 120 (day two of cycle)

PRL—200

TSH—1.2

Testosterone—0.8

USS—NAD

HSG—Patent tubes

Rubella immune

Chlamydia swabs—ve

Smear—ve

Semen analysis—10m/ml, 32% motility, 3% normal forms

Ask them if they want to arrange any further investigations.

Expect candidate to ask to repeat gonadotrophins more than a month after initial measurement in order to confirm the diagnosis of Premature Ovarian Insufficiency (POI). They should also repeat the semen analysis.

Tell them that repeat gonadotrophins were again elevated—FSH 35, LH 20, E2 120. Repeat semen analysis was 15m/ml, 34% motile, with 4% normal forms.

Ask the candidate to explain these results to the patient and explain next steps, including further investigation and treatment options.

They should then recommend that further investigations are arranged including karyotype, an autoimmune screen, lupus anticoagulant and vitamin B12 levels to try and identify a cause for the POI. Treatment options should include the role of hormone replacement therapy and oocyte donation with IVF.

Observe consultation skills including the candidate's ability to break bad news.

Record your overall clinical impression of the candidate for each domain (i.e. pass, borderline, or fail).

Instructions for Role Player

You are Janet Jones, aged 28 years, and have been trying to conceive for around two years. Your cycle used to be regular but over the past year has become increasingly irregular with a cycle length varying between 35 and 60 days. Your last period was 50 days ago. You have put on some weight in this last year and wonder if this is responsible.

If asked—you have never had any operations or pelvic infections, are not on any medication and have no allergies. You are immune to rubella. You do not report headaches, visual disturbance, galactorrhoea, or acne and hirsutism. However, you have noticed that you feel tired and rather irritable and feel hot at night. You do not smoke.

Your partner, Peter, had an orchidopexy at the age of two. He is also not on any medication, nor does he smoke.

Concerns: You are worried that you are not ovulating and are frightened that this is an early menopause (your mother had her menopause at 40). You really want to get pregnant and give up your job, which you dislike (shelf stacker at local supermarket).

Expectations: You expect the doctor to find out why your periods are irregular and if this is preventing you from becoming pregnant.

When told that you have premature ovarian insufficiency you are upset and become more so if the doctor explains this poorly and/or is not empathetic.

You want to know what treatment you could have.

Assessment

Marking Scheme

Patient safety:

Pass Borderline Fail

Communication with patients and their relatives:

Pass Borderline Fail

Information gathering:

Pass Borderline Fail

Applied clinical knowledge:

Pass Borderline Fail

Notes for Marking

Patient safety

- Assesses the patients' main concerns
- Identifies appropriate investigations to make a diagnosis
- Is aware of risks of proposed treatment
- Explains that treatment will depend on the outcome of her final tests

Communication with patients and their relatives

- Greets, introduces self and role, and checks patients' names
- Breaks bad news sensitively—premature ovarian insufficiency
- Uses appropriate communication skills (chunking and checking, summarising, checking understanding)
- Addresses patient's concerns and expectations

Information gathering

- Key points of clinical history and results
- Open and honest about the diagnosis and its implications

Applied clinical knowledge

- Aetiology of oligo- and amenorrhoea
- Knows appropriate investigations for subfertility and oligomenorrhoea and can interpret these
- Diagnosis of POI and further investigations required to identify possible causes

Notes for Candidates

It is important that you summarize and interpret results of investigations and
Present a clear and logical plan for further investigation and management to assessor.

Further reading

Management of women with premature ovarian insufficiency Guideline of the European Society of Human Reproduction and Embryology, December 2015. https://www.eshre.eu/.../Guidelines/.../ESHRE-guideline_POI-2015_FINAL_1112201

Task 2 **Anovulatory infertility (cont'd)**

Instructions for candidate

This task assesses the following clinical skills:

- Patient safety
- Communication with patients and their relatives
- Information gathering
- Applied clinical knowledge

The same couple have returned to the clinic. The consultant is away. Karyotype has come back as XO/XX with small amount of XY (Turner mosaic).

Explain this result to the patient and plan further management with them.

You have 10 minutes for this task (+ 2mins initial reading time).

Instructions for Assessors

Please read instructions to candidate and actor.

Allow candidate to explain Turner syndrome to the patient. Expect them to discuss further investigations and need for a gonadectomy (XY component) and long term monitoring. They should explain that it is important to assess cardiac function (MRI) in advance of considering using donor oocytes to conceive.

Record your overall clinical impression of the candidate for each domain (i.e. pass, borderline, or fail).

Instructions for Role Players

Please see clinical assessment task 16.2 'Instructions for the role players' for background.

You were upset to learn at your last consultation that your ovaries were not working properly. You do not understand what being a Turner mosaic means and want the doctor to explain this to you. You have never heard of this condition before.

You have looked up premature menopause on the internet and know that you could use donor eggs via an IVF process to get pregnant. You want to know if you can do this as you are still very keen to start a family—although you are beginning to despair about this.

Assessment

Marking Scheme

Patient safety:

Pass Borderline Fail

Communication with patients and their relatives:

Pass Borderline Fail

Information gathering:

Pass Borderline Fail

Applied clinical knowledge:

Pass Borderline Fail

Notes for Marking

Patient safety

- Assesses the patients' main concerns
- Identifies appropriate investigations to make a diagnosis
- Is aware of risks of proposed treatment
- Explains that treatment will depend on the outcome of her final tests

Communication with patients and their relatives

- Greets, introduces self and role, and checks patients' names
- Breaks bad news sensitively—premature ovarian insufficiency
- Uses appropriate communication skills (chunking and checking, summarizing, checking understanding)
- Addresses patient's concerns and expectations

Information gathering

- Key points of clinical history and results
- Open and honest about the diagnosis and its implications

Applied clinical knowledge

- Aetiology of oligo- and amenorrhoea
- Knows appropriate investigations for subfertility and oligomenorrhoea and can interpret these
- Diagnosis of POI and further investigations required to identify possible causes

Notes for Candidates

It is important that you summarize and interpret results of investigations and

Present a clear and logical plan for further investigation and management to the assessor.

Anovulatory infertility has been classified by the WHO into three groups. Group 1 is hypothalamic pituitary failure (low gonadotrophins and low oestrogen). Group 2 is hypothalamic pituitary dysfunction (e.g. PCOS) and group 3 is ovarian failure or insufficiency (POI) (high gonadotrophins and low oestrogen).

Although POI is rare in this age group, the diagnosis is sometimes made during investigations for infertility and is confirmed by finding elevated gonadotrophins (with low oestrogen) on two occasions at least a month apart. Although the cause is often not identified further investigations should exclude genetic and auto immune conditions, lupus, vitamin B12 deficiency and galactosemia. POI may also result from chemo or radiotherapy following an oncological diagnosis. Treatment includes hormone replacement therapy (patients may occasionally ovulate spontaneously on treatment) and oocyte donation with IVF. Turner syndrome (usually mosaicism in this context) is a rare but important genetic cause and all patients with POI should have a karyotype checked. Turner syndrome is a multisystem disorder—patients need screening for cardiac, renal, liver and thyroid dysfunction, coeliac disease and auditory problems. It is important to refer them to a cardiologist to exclude cardiac disease if they are contemplating pregnancy via oocyte donation as maternal deaths have been recorded. Single embryo transfer is recommended as these patients have high risk pregnancies.

Patients with other causes of their anovulation may be suitable for ovulation induction with either clomifene (an anti-oestrogen) or gonadotrophins. The former is appropriate for patients with an intact HPO axis (WHO group 2) as first line therapy. Gonadotrophins are used when clomifene has failed, or as first line treatment when the pituitary cannot produce LH and FSH (WHO group 1). Pulsatile gonadotrophin releasing hormone can also successfully induce unifollicular ovulation in patients in

WHO group 1 who have an intact pituitary. Underweight patients should be encouraged to put on weight as first line therapy. Hyperprolactinaemia is treated with dopamine agonists (bromocriptine or cabergoline). Laparoscopic ovarian diathermy has been used in patients with PCOS.

The main complications of treatment are multiple pregnancy and ovarian hyperstimulation (OHSS). The latter is a particular risk for patients with PCOS. These risks should be explained to patients embarking on ovulation induction. Both of these complications can be reduced or avoided by careful planning of treatment and monitoring.

Notes on subfertility

Subfertility is usually defined as an inability to conceive for a year. However, this definition can vary depending on the patient's age, cycle length or past history. It is common—some studies suggest that one in seven couples will have problems conceiving. The main reasons for subfertility are anovulation, tubal damage and male factor. If investigations fail to demonstrate any abnormality, infertility is described as being unexplained. Appropriate treatment is dependent on identifying the cause of the subfertility.

Partners are seen together in clinics which can make the consultation more challenging as histories need to be taken from both and appropriate examination and investigation arranged—also for both. Currently commissioning groups around the UK variably fund assisted conception, which adds further complexity to discussions with patients about suitable treatment.

Anovulatory subfertility

Around 20% of primary and 15% of secondary infertility is caused by anovulation. Causes can be classified according to the site of dysfunction on the hypothalamic –pituitary-ovarian axis. Hypothalamic causes include weight loss, excessive exercise, stress, tumours, and Kallman's syndrome. Pituitary causes include tumours, hyperprolactinaemia, radiotherapy, surgery, empty sella syndrome and rarely nowadays necrosis following major post partum haemorrhage (Sheehan's syndrome). Ovarian insufficiency or failure may result from genetic causes (for example, Turner syndrome), auto-immunity, or may be iatrogenic following surgery, chemo or radiotherapy. Polycystic ovaries cause dysfunction of the hypothalamic—pituitary-ovarian axis. Other causes include chronic disease and thyroid dysfunction.

Key knowledge:

- Hypothalamic pituitary ovarian axis
- Hormone changes in menstrual and ovarian cycles
- Aetiology of anovulation
- Appropriate investigation of anovulation
- Available treatment including clomifene and gonadotrophin ovulation induction. Role of In vitro fertilization (IVF).
- Complications of treatment including multiple pregnancy and ovarian hyperstimulation syndrome (OHSS)

Key skills

- Consultation with couple—information gathering, explanation and planning
- Interpretation of results

In anovulatory subfertility, clinical assessment tasks may include history taking, planning investigation, analysing results and identifying the cause of anovulation. They may also involve discussion of appropriate treatment with a couple including an exploration of risks and complications.

Further reading

Bhattacharya S, Hamilton M, eds. *Management of infertility for the MRCOG and beyond.* 3rd edition. 2014. Cambridge: Cambridge University Press.

Balen A. *Infertility in practice*. 3rd edition. 2008 Elsevier Press.

Yasmin E, Davies M, Conway G, Balen AH. 'Ovulation induction in WHO Type 1 anovulation: Guidelines for practice'. Produced on behalf of the BFS Policy and Practice Committee. 2013. British Fertility Society. *Hum Fertil*, 16(4) 228–34.

Task 3 **Tubal factor infertility**

Instructions for Candidate

This task assesses the following clinical skills:

- Patient safety
- Communication with patients and their relatives
- Information gathering
- Applied clinical knowledge

You are an ST5 doctor helping your consultant in the reproductive medicine clinic. Your consultant has asked you to see a couple coming for a return consultation after additional testing for primary subfertility. You quickly look at the results, ovulation is confirmed and semen analysis is normal, but the HSG shows a unilateral hydrosalpinx without spill. The consultant asked you to explain to the couple that she would propose a laparoscopy. Please explain to the couple the implications of the test results and the treatment plan.

After the consultation you will be given the laparoscopy findings and asked some questions by the assessor.

You have 10 minutes for this task (+ 2mins initial reading time).

Instructions for Assessor

Please read instructions to candidate and actor.

Allow the candidate to conduct the interview undisturbed unless they are straying off the track of the question (in which case you can show them their instructions again).

This patient has tubal subfertility; the consultation should cover:

- Laparoscopy
- Previous surgery
- Explanation of tubal occlusion

Once the candidate has taken a relevant history and presented to you, provide the candidate with the following information:

- Laparoscopy was performed and showed Fitz-Hugh Curtis adhesions, the occluded tube was removed and the contralateral tube looked normal and could be preserved

Now ask the candidate to explain the most likely diagnosis of previous PID to Lauren.

Lauren is worried that the HSG has caused the adhesions, please address that.

Record your overall clinical impression of the candidate for each domain (e.g. should this performance be pass, borderline, or a fail).

Instructions for Role Player

You are Lauren Pitt, aged 32. You are married to James. You have been trying to get pregnant for over two years. You both work for the University. You have had multiple boyfriends during your studies. At the moment all is set up for starting your family.

If you are specifically asked:

- You never had STI tests before your fertility referral by your GP
- You have had some courses of antibiotics during your twenties because of recurrent tonsillitis

- Before starting to try you have used the combined pill
- Your family history is non-significant
- You do not have pelvic pain
- Your cycles are regular
- No problems with cervical smears
- You did not have your appendix removed

Temperament: You think you are an analytical person. You like numbers and figures. You do not like hospitals and are afraid of needles.

Ideas: You were expecting that everything would be normal. Bad things happen to other people. You are expecting the doctor to tell you that you need to continue trying and will get pregnant without treatment. You are not expecting surgery.

Concerns: You are scared to have an operation, and want to find out more about laparoscopy.

Expectations: You want the doctor to explain the following:

- Alternative to laparoscopy
- The procedure itself
- Risks and benefits associated with the procedure
- Who will be doing it?
- What happens if there are complications? What is the chance of anything going wrong during your operation?
- Can anything be done to reduce the chance of having any complication?
- When can you go back to work?

Assessment

Marking Scheme

Patient safety:

Pass Borderline Fail

Communication with patients and their relatives:

Pass Borderline Fail

Information gathering:

Pass Borderline Fail

Applied clinical knowledge:

Pass Borderline Fail

Notes for Marking

Patient safety

- Assesses the patient's main concerns and ideas
- Gives options and discusses the pros and cons of Laparoscopy
- Discusses possible complications and measures to reduce them
- Involves patient in the process (e.g. encouraging them to express their ideas, or preferences)
- Negotiates a mutually agreed acceptable, safe, plan

- Open and honest about procedure and possible complications
- Provides with information about the possibility of finding a normal pelvis due to tubal spasm during the HSG

Communication with patients and their relatives

- Greets, introduces self and role, checks patient's name
- Consent to proceed and explains nature of interview
- Assesses patient's starting point (what the patient wants to know) and sets the agenda
- Clear organized explanation in logical sequence
- Chunks: e.g. provides information in reasonable chunks
- Checks patient understands.
- Language (easily understood, avoids or explains jargon)
- Uses visual aids appropriately e.g. diagrams or uses analogies to aid explanation
- Presents a clear and succinct history to the assessor

Information gathering

- Key points of clinical history and results.
- Open and honest about the diagnosis and its implications

Applied clinical knowledge

- Demonstrates a sound and comprehensive evidence-based clinical knowledge—e.g. confirms standard practice and reiterates laparoscopy as gold standard test for tubal subfertility. Counsel the patient about removing hydrosalpinx before IVF. Explain the increase risk of ectopic pregnancy
- Justify management plan

Notes for Candidate

The scenario is taken from a common clinical scenario of our daily practice. It not only assesses the process of communication but also assesses the content of the knowledge given to the patient. It is important how you provide the information to the patient.

Practice this scenario with one of your friends who can act as a role player and ask another friend to provide you with feedback. We recommend you read the following: Fertility problems: assessment and treatment NICE guideline.

Chlamydia trachomatis

- Present in 11% of the sexually active population aged 19 years or less
- Major cause of pelvic inflammatory disease, leading to chronic abdominal pain, ectopic pregnancy and tubal factor infertility
- Asymptomatic chlamydial infection may go unrecognized and untreated
- Prevalence of C. trachomatis among subfertile women in the UK is only 1.9%
- Uterine instrumentation carried out routinely as part of the infertility investigation may reactivate or introduce upper tract dissemination of endocervical chlamydial infection
- Clinical pelvic infection following hysterosalpingography (HSG) has been reported in up to 4% of cases and in 10% of patients with tubal disease

Assessing tubal damage

- Tubal factors account for 14% of the causes of subfertility in women
- Proximal (uterotubal) obstruction occurs in 10–25% of women with tubal disease
- An ideal (or 'gold standard') test for tubal disease would correctly identify all women with tubal disease

Hysterosalpingography compared with laparoscopy and dye.

HSG and laparoscopy with dye are the two most widely used methods to test for tubal pathology. HSG and laparoscopy are both invasive procedures but HSG is less so. Among women whose tubes were found to be patent (unobstructed) using HSG, 18% were found to have tubal obstruction or peritubal adhesions using laparoscopy.

The diagnostic accuracy of HSG has been compared with that of laparoscopy and dye in a meta-analysis pooled estimates of sensitivity and specificity for HSG as a test for tubal obstruction of 0.65 (95% CI 0.50 to 0.78) and 0.83 (95% CI 0.77 to 0.88), respectively. It is estimated that tubal damage accounts for 14% of fertility problems, which suggests that when HSG suggests the presence of tubal obstruction this will be confirmed by laparoscopy in only 38% of women.

Thus, HSG is a not a reliable indicator of tubal occlusion. However, when HSG suggests that the tubes are patent, this will be confirmed at laparoscopy in 94% of women, and so HSG is a reliable indicator of tubal patency.

Results from another review suggest that HSG could be used as a screening test for couples with no history of pelvic infection, and if abnormal, confirmatory laparoscopy would follow.

Hysterosalpingo-contrast-sonography compared with laparoscopy and dye or hysterosalpingography.

Evaluative studies of hysterosalpingo-contrast-sonogaphy (HyCoSy) showed good statistical comparability and concordance with HSG and laparoscopy combined with dye. HyCoSy is well-tolerated and can be a suitable alternative outpatient procedure.

Tubal flushing

The potential therapeutic effect of diagnostic tubal patency testing has been debated for over 40 years. Tubal flushing might involve water- or oil-soluble media. Current practice usually involves water-soluble media when tubal flushing is performed at laparoscopy. A systematic review of eight RCTs showed a significant increase in pregnancy rates with tubal flushing using oil-soluble contrast media when compared with no treatment (OR 3.57, 95% CI 1.76 to 7.23). Tubal flushing with oil-soluble contrast media was associated with an increase in the odds of live birth (OR 1.49, 95% CI 1.05 to 2.11), but not pregnancy rates (OR 1.23, 95% CI 0.95 to 1.60) when compared with tubal flushing with water-soluble media. There were no significant differences in miscarriage, ectopic pregnancy and infection rates between tubal flushing with oil or water, or between oil plus water media versus water media only. There were no trials assessing tubal flushing with water-soluble media versus no treatment.

The potential consequences of extravasations of oil-soluble contrast media into the pelvic cavity and fallopian tubes may be associated with anaphylaxis and lipogranuloma.

Further reading

Fertility problems: assessment and treatment Clinical guideline [CG156] February 2013 Last updated August 2016. https://www.nice.org.uk/guidance/cg156?unlid=46855266201611595632

Task 4 **PCOS**

Instructions for Candidate

This task assesses the following clinical skills:

- Patient safety
- Communication with patients and their relatives
- Information gathering
- Applied clinical knowledge

Francesca Bulthorpe is a 32-year-old lady with a BMI of 48. She has irregular periods, hirsutism and has been diagnosed with polycystic ovarian syndrome by the Rotterdam criteria.

In spite of previous counselling and referral to weight management, Francesca has not made any progress regarding her weight management, often not attending the weight management sessions.

Your consultant has therefore asked you to explain to Francesca:

- What does PCOS mean
- Counsel regarding the long term implications of PCOS on her health
- Counsel regarding the positive effects of life-style modification

You have 10 minutes for this task (+ 2mins initial reading time).

Instructions for Assessor

This clinical assessment task assesses the candidate's ability to explain in a logical, non-patronizing manner, the condition of PCOS, its long term implications and the positive impact of life style modification.

If the candidate starts to skirt around the problem, the role player will interrupt. This clinical assessment task also assesses the candidate's ability to deal with such a scenario.

Instructions for Role Player

You are Francesca Bultorpe, a 32-year-old, working as a prison guard.

You are in a same sex relationship. You have been with your partner for the last seven years. Your partner is slim.

You have always been a big girl. Both your mother and sister are big as well. Your father died of a heart attack when you were nine years old.

You have suffered with heavy and irregular periods which have now been controlled with a progesterone medicated coil. You have excess facial and lower abdominal hair.

You have been told to reduce weight, but do not understand what the fuss is all about. In your job, it is not always bad to appear big. If at all you and your partner decide to have a baby, it will be her becoming pregnant as she is a teacher and has a regular nine to five job.

Yes, you are bothered by the excess hair, but do not see how decreasing weight is going to affect that.

Temperament: You are generally calm but you are an impatient person and do not like conversations where people beat around the bush rather than come to the point. You are likely to interrupt the conversation if that happens.

Ideas: You just want your consultant and his team to treat the periods, which they have and leave you alone. You cannot see how having PCOS is going to have any impact on your health.

Concerns: You are concerned that every visit, you are lectured on the importance of weight loss. You cannot see how it is going to reduce your excess facial hair. You also feel that this condition of PCOS is making you put on weight.

You are concerned that you will be made to listen to another session on how to reduce your weight.

Expectations: Your expectation is that the doctor you are about to talk to, talks to the point, and if wants to encourage weight reduction, motivates you by explaining the relevance

Assessment

Marking Scheme

Patient safety:

Pass Borderline Fail

Communication with patients and their relatives:

Pass Borderline Fail

Information gathering:

Pass Borderline Fail

Applied clinical knowledge:

Pass Borderline Fail

Notes for Marking

Patient safety

- Assesses the patient's main concerns and ideas
- Elicits patients ideas, concerns and expectation and relates explanations to these
- Shows interest and respect, empathizes and supports patient (expresses understanding, concern and willingness to help)
- Open and honest about long term health implications

Communication with patients and their relatives

- Consent to proceed and explains nature of interview
- Assesses patient's starting point (what the patient wants to know) and sets the agenda
- Clear organized explanation e.g. small chunks in logical sequence
- Checks patient's understanding Full marks if does this more than once and gets patient to repeat in their own words
- Screens appropriately e.g. 'Is there something else?'
- Language (easily understood, avoids or explains jargon)
- Uses visual aids appropriately e.g. diagrams or uses analogies to aid explanation
- Sign-posting e.g. 'there are three things I'd like to discuss, first ... then ....'
- Summarizes at intervals to clarify what has been said

Information gathering

- Key points of clinical history and results
- Open and honest about the diagnosis and its implications

Applied clinical knowledge

- Demonstrates a sound and comprehensive evidence-based clinical knowledge
- Counsels the patient with relevant information that is factually correct
- Explains PCOS in a way that the patient will understand. May use diagrams, e.g. for explanation—polycystic ovaries contain a large number of harmless follicles that are up to 8mm (approximately 0.3in) in size. The follicles are under-developed sacs in which eggs develop. In PCOS, these sacs are often unable to release an egg, which means that ovulation doesn't take place
- Explanation regarding the cause, e.g.—the exact cause of PCOS is unknown, but it often runs in families. It's related to abnormal hormone levels in the body, including high levels of insulin. Insulin is a hormone that controls sugar levels in the body. Many women with PCOS are resistant to the action of insulin in their body and produce higher levels of insulin to overcome this. This contributes to the increased production and activity of hormones such as testosterone. Being overweight or obese also increases the amount of insulin your body produces
- That there is no strong evidence that PCOS by itself can cause weight gain or that having PCOS makes weight loss difficult or impossible
- Should counsel regarding Diabetes and offer screening for Type 2 diabetes
- Counsel regarding the high risk of cardiovascular disease and all women with PCOS should be assessed for CVD risk by assessing individual CVD risk factors (obesity, lack of physical activity, cigarette smoking, family history of Type 2 diabetes, dyslipidaemia, hypertension, impaired glucose tolerance, Type 2 diabetes) at the time of initial diagnosis
- Oligo- or amenorrhoea in women with PCOS may predispose to endometrial hyperplasia and later carcinoma. However, Francesca should be reassured that the progesterone coil is helping protect the lining of the womb
- Now, explain how weight reduction will help reduce the insulin resistance and therefore help reduce the risk of diabetes and cardiovascular disease
- Explains the importance of both diet and exercise
- Explains the possibility of bariatric surgery, given Francescas very high BMI and familial risk factors

Further reading

Long-term Consequences of Polycystic Ovary Syndrome Green-top Guideline No. 33 November 2014. https://www.rcog.org.uk/globalassets/documents/guidelines/gtg_33.pdf

Task 5 **OHSS**

Instructions for Candidate

This task assesses the following clinical skills:

- Patient safety
- Communication with patients and their relatives
- Information gathering
- Applied clinical knowledge

You are an ST4 doctor holding the bleep for gynae. You are bleeped by the doctor from A & E asking you to review Yvi Fonderson. Please take a brief history and tell her what your most likely diagnosis is. You do not need to examine her. Once you have completed taking the history you will be asked to give a brief summary of the relevant points in the history and differential diagnosis to the assessor.

You will be given the examination findings and asked some questions by the assessor.

You have 10 minutes for this task (+ 2mins initial reading time).

Instructions for Assessor

Please read instructions to candidate and actor.

Allow the candidate to conduct the interview undisturbed unless they are straying off the track of the question (in which case you can show them their instructions again).

This patient has late onset OHSS. The history should cover:

- Start and duration of symptoms
- Presence of dyspnoea, abdominal distension, abdominal pain, nausea, and vomiting
- Urine output
- She should be informed that mild forms of OHSS are common, affecting up to 33% of fertilization (IVF) cycles and that 3–8% of IVF cycles are complicated by moderate or severe OHSS
- Exclude ovarian torsion
- Exclude pelvic infection
- PMH and PSH, family history, social history and current drug history
- IVF history

Once the candidate has taken a relevant history and presented to you, provide the candidate with the following information:

- Abdominal examination—distended abdomen, mildly tender, shifting dullness
- Trans-abdominal and Trans-vaginal scan
  - Transvaginal scan was carried out with verbal consent
  - Uterus in anteverted flexion, Endometrial thickness 12mm, the endometrium was clearly visualized
  - Both ovaries are enlarged containing multiple follicular cysts, maximal diameter of ovaries is 7cm
  - 4cm of free fluid in the pouch of Douglas
- Lab: Hb 150, Hct 0.45, platelets 350, normal renal and liver function tests

Plan: For outpatient management.

Now ask the candidate to explain the management plan to Mrs J Wright

There are some marks on the process mark sheet for the actor to assign at the end of the station.

Record your overall clinical impression of the candidate for each domain (e.g. should this performance be pass, borderline, or a fail).

Instructions for Role Player

You are Yvi Fonderson, aged 28. You are married to Ashley. You have been together for seven years.

Ashley has poor sperm quality due to testicular surgery as a child. You have just had your first round of IVF. You had an embryo transfer ten days ago. You are due to do a urine pregnancy test in four days. You are not feeling well, after contacting your local IVF unit, you were advice to go to Accident and Emergency Department. You are off your food and find it difficult to sleep.

If you are specifically asked:

- You had one embryo in the day five stage transfer
- You started feeling unwell five days ago
- They collected 21 eggs
- Your cannot lay flat on your back without getting short of breath
- You are passing urine, but it looks dark
- When you are resting you have no problems breathing
- You have been sick once, and feel a little nauseated but you are able to eat small meals
- You are taking progesterone supplementation, you are scared to take paracetamol
- The IVF unit did say that you had high hormone levels, but you are unsure what they were
- You cannot wear your normal jeans and have been wearing loose dresses
- You have a normal menstrual cycle and have never been diagnosed with PCOS
- Your BMI is 20
- You do not have a fever
- You have generalized abdominal pain coming on and off
- No bleeding
- No diarrhoea

Temperament: You think you are a calm, level-headed woman. You value information as you can get anxious about the possibility of not becoming a mother. The IVF process has made you more emotional.

Ideas: You were expecting blood tests and to be told that this is all normal with IVF. You were not expecting hospitalization.

Concerns: You are worried about a potential pregnancy. You do not want Ashley to worry as he feels it is his entire fault. You do not want to take time off work as they do not know about the fertility treatment. You want to know what is happening and if there are any risks for you and the baby.

Expectations: You want the doctor to explain the following:

- What is happening to you—what is hyperstimulation?
- When will it stop?
- Could it have been predicted?
- What additional tests will be done?
- What can you do to improve symptoms?
- What are the risks associated with OHSS?
- What is the risk for the outcome of the pregnancy?

Assessment

Marking Scheme

Patient safety:

Pass	Borderline	Fail

Communication with patients and their relatives:

Pass	Borderline	Fail

Information gathering:

Pass	Borderline	Fail

Applied clinical knowledge:

Pass	Borderline	Fail

Notes for Marking

Patient safety

- Assesses the patient's main concerns and ideas. Explains to continue with the progesterone, and do the pregnancy test as planned. Explained that a blood pregnancy test can still be false positive after the ovarian stimulation. A pregnancy is likely, but it is too early to confirm
- Discusses possible complications and measures to reduce them
- Involves patient in the process (e.g. encouraging them to express their ideas, or preferences)
- Negotiates a mutually agreed acceptable, safe, plan
- Open and honest about diagnosis and possible complications
- Provides with information about the syndrome and follow-up
- Explain mechanism in place to deal with problems out of hours
- Informing HFEA, performing IVF unit

Communication with patients and their relatives

- Greets, introduces self and role, checks patient's name
- Consent to proceed and explains nature of interview
- Assesses patient's starting point (what the patient wants to know) and sets the agenda
- Clear organized explanation in logical sequence
- Chunks: e.g. provides information in reasonable chunks
- Checks patient's understanding.
- Language (easily understood, avoids or explains jargon)
- Uses visual aids appropriately e.g. diagrams or uses analogies to aid explanation
- Presents a clear and succinct history to the assessor

Information gathering

- Key points of clinical history and results.
- Open and honest about the diagnosis and its implications

Applied clinical knowledge

- Demonstrates a sound and comprehensive evidence-based clinical knowledge—e.g. confirms the diagnosis of OHSS. Counsels the patient with relevant information that is factually correct (risks of ARDS, thrombosis)
- Discusses management as out or inpatient. Justify management plan

Notes for Candidate

The scenario is taken from a common clinical scenario of our daily practice. It not only assesses the process of communication but also assesses the content of the knowledge given to the patient. It is important how you provide the information to the patient.

Practice this scenario with one of your friends who can act as a role player and ask another friend to provide you with feedback.

We recommend you read the RCOG guideline. Here is a summary of some of the most important points:

- Treatment for women with mild OHSS and many with moderate OHSS can be managed on an outpatient basis
- Analgesia using paracetamol or codeine is appropriate. Nonsteroidal anti-inflammatory drugs should not be used
- Women should be encouraged to drink to thirst, rather than to excess.
- Strenuous exercise and sexual intercourse should be avoided for fear of injury or torsion of hyperstimulated ovaries
- Women should continue progesterone luteal support but HCG luteal support is inappropriate
- Counselling support for both the woman and her partner provides reassurance and information to allay anxiety

Assessment of the woman will usually involve clinical examination, which should include body weight and abdominal girth measurement, and pelvic ultrasound examination to measure ovarian size and check for ascites. Laboratory investigations that are helpful in assessing the severity of OHSS are haemoglobin, haematocrit, serum creatinine and electrolytes and liver function tests. Baseline values may help track the progress of the condition.

Review every two to three days is likely to be adequate. However, urgent clinical review is necessary if the woman develops increasing severity of pain, increasing abdominal distension shortness of breath and a subjective impression of reduced urine output. If the woman conceives, prolonged monitoring may be appropriate.

Women with severe OHSS require inpatient management. In addition, women with moderate OHSS who are unable to achieve control of their pain and/or nausea with oral treatment should also be admitted. Admission should also be considered where there are difficulties in ensuring adequate ongoing monitoring, until resolution commences.

The reported incidence of thrombosis with OHSS ranges between 0.7% and 10%, with an apparent preponderance of upper body sites and frequent involvement of the arterial system.

Women should be reassured that pregnancy may continue normally despite OHSS, and there is no evidence of an increased risk of congenital abnormalities.

Further reading

The management of Ovarian Hyperstimulation Syndrome Green-to Guideline No 6; RCOG; February 2016. https://www.rcog.org.uk/globalassets/documents/guidelines/green-top-guidelines/gtg_5_ohss.pdf

Chapter 16 **Sexual and Reproductive Health**

Task 1 **Contraception**

Instructions for Candidate

This task assesses the following clinical skills:

- Patient safety
- Communication with patients and their relatives
- Information gathering
- Applied clinical knowledge

You are an ST4 doctor conducting a post operative ward round. Your next patient is Danielle Wilson, a 26-year-old mother of three who has undergone a left salpingectomy for ectopic pregnancy. Having explained the operation to her, she asks why you couldn't have just sterilized her at the same time as she never wants to be pregnant again and is struggling with her health and her young children. Her notes show that she has had 2 previous terminations and takes carbamazepine and levetiracetam for epilepsy and fluoxetine for anxiety. There is nothing else of note.

Explain to Danielle why she was not sterilized at the time of salpingectomy. Then make a safe and effective contraception plan which is acceptable to her.

You have 10 minutes for this task (+ 2mins initial reading time).

Instruction for Assessor

Ask the candidate and actor to read their instructions. Then ask the candidate to start their discussion with the patient.

Allow the candidate to conduct the discussion undisturbed unless they are straying off the track of the question (in which case you can show them their instructions again).

Rationale for not sterilising should cover

- General inadvisability of performing procedure at a time of reproductive stress (e.g. delivery, termination of pregnancy [TOP], miscarriage, salpingectomy)
- Sterilization under age 30 associated with higher incidence of regret—this should be conveyed as a general rule of thumb rather than as a personal judgement
- Reversal not funded by NHS
- Higher failure rate when performed when pregnant
- Possible complications of sterilization—general anaesthetic, surgical trauma or if hysteroscopic day case procedure, uterine perforation, interval to confirmation of success, need for ongoing contraceptive method
- Lifetime failure rate of sterilisation 1:200 which is comparable to that of an IUS and higher than the failure rate of the contraceptive implant
- Vasectomy safer

Choice of other contraceptive methods

- Could use a method until over age 30 years, when a request for sterilization may be looked on more favourably
- Contraindicated—oral contraception (both combined and progestogen only) and sub dermal implant—because of enzyme inducer CARBAMAZEPINE
- Not contraindicated—contraceptive injection and intrauterine methods (IUS and IUD)
- Patient preference of methods which are suitable –not injection as terrified of needles. Uncertain of IUD/IUS because worried that they are harmful
- The candidate should elicit her reservations, recognize that the injection is unacceptable to her and explore further the possibility of intrauterine methods including reliability, some discomfort during insertion, user independence, and long acting method, no increased risk of sexually transmitted infections and lighter bleeds or amenorrhoea with an IUS
- Explain that IUS amenorrhoea is not harmful

Plan: Danielle should be signposted to her GP or the Contraception & Sexual Health Service for IUS insertion. Written information on the method and condoms until then can be offered.

There are some marks on the process mark sheet for the actor to assign at the end of the station.

Record your overall clinical impression of the candidate for each domain (e.g. should this performance be pass, borderlin,e or a fail).

Instructions for Role Player

You are Danielle Wilson, aged 26. You are a single mother with an on/off partner who is the father of the youngest two of your children. Your children are aged ten, five and three. Your eldest child, a son called Jordan has ADHD which is very challenging. You had a termination of pregnancy in the year after he was born. Your younger two children were unplanned and you had a second termination of pregnancy a year ago.

You have been using condoms and withdrawal for contraception and were shocked to find out you were pregnant this time as you were being careful. Your partner doesn't help much at home, doesn't like using condoms and wouldn't consider vasectomy.

You were even more upset to be told you had a life threatening ectopic pregnancy requiring emergency surgery and frustrated at the refusal to sterilize you at the same time simply because you are 'too young'.

You are very anxious about the future and your ability to cope with your children, your seizures and your mental health.

Your preferences for contraception: Sterilization is your preferred method. You do not associate it with any harmful side effects or a failure rate. You are more likely to consider a contraceptive method if you are told that sterilization can result in surgical complications, actually has a failure rate and that you could perhaps have the procedure when over 30 and use something else as a shorter term measure.

Contraceptive pills: If asked about pills you will say that you had them in the past but fell pregnant on them anyway and don't trust them. You also know that they might interact with your epilepsy medication since it was changed last time and you will query this if pills are discussed.

Contraceptive implant or injection: You hate needles and won't consider these.

Intrauterine device or system (coil): Initially hesitant as you think they are painful to insert and cause damage and infection. If you are told there is only a very small risk of perforation and that insertion, although uncomfortable, is tolerable, particularly when balanced against five or ten years use, you may start to consider this option until you can be sterilized. You like the idea of lighter or absent periods (with the Mirena IUS/hormone coil), but wonder if it is harmful to have no periods at all?

Expectations: A clear and non-patronizing explanation of your options, taking your needle phobia into account and your desire to have something really effective, will help you feel much less frustrated and more in control of your future.

Assessment

Marking Scheme

Patient safety:

Pass	Borderline	Fail

Communication with patients and their relatives:

Pass	Borderline	Fail

Information gathering:

Pass	Borderline	Fail

Applied clinical knowledge:

Pass	Borderline	Fail

Notes for Marking

Applied clinical knowledge

- Demonstrates a sound and comprehensive evidence-based clinical knowledge—counsels the patient with relevant information that is factually correct e.g. sterilization is not usually performed at the time of delivery, miscarriage, termination, or salpingectomy for ectopic pregnancy, higher instance of regret under age 30 years, risks associated with laparoscopic approach and hysteroscopic approach, lifetime failure rate
- Discusses alternative management plan e.g. contraception until a bit older when sterilization may be performed

Communication with patients and their relatives and colleagues

- Greets, introduces self and role, checks patient's name and explains nature of interview
- Assesses patient's starting point (what the patient wants to know) and sets the agenda. Listens to preferences
- Clear organized explanation in logical sequence
- Chunks: e.g. provides information in reasonable chunks
- Checks patient's understanding.
- Language (easily understood, avoids or explains jargon)
- Uses visual aids appropriately e.g. diagrams or uses analogies to aid explanation
- Involves patient in the process (e.g. encouraging them to express their ideas, or preferences
- Negotiates a mutually agreed, acceptable, safe plan

Patient safety and quality

- Assesses the patient's main concerns and ideas
- Differentiate between methods that are contraindicated and/or completely unacceptable to the patient and those which may be acceptable after further discussion
- Gives options and discusses the risks and benefits of intrauterine methods

Maintaining trust

- Explains information in a non-patronizing, objective way
- Acknowledges the many difficulties that this patient faces and uses this as a starting point for planning the most effective (and convenient) contraceptive method

Notes for Candidate

This scenario is about making a contraceptive plan with a woman who would prefer sterilization but is not an ideal candidate because of her young age. In order to be effective, the candidate should acknowledge the patient's frustration at being refused what she wants and try to formulate a compromize solution with her. Clarity, objectivity and a woman centred (non-paternalistic) communication style are essential in order to gain rapport in this scenario.

Further reading

Clinical Guidance: Drug Interactions with Hormonal Contraception. Jan 2017. www.fsrh.org
Contraception Made Easy by Laura Percy and Diana Mansour

Task 2 **Contraceptive implant**

Instructions for Candidate

This task assesses the following clinical skills:

- Patient safety
- Communication with patients and their relatives
- Information gathering
- Applied clinical knowledge

You are an ST-4 Doctor working in a gynaecologycClinic with your consultant. Your Consultant asks you to see Mrs Julie Smith who has been referred by her GP for counselling for the contraceptive implant.

Your task is to:

- Assess her suitability for the contraceptive implant
- Counsel her regarding the issues relevant to the contraceptive implant
- Answer her questions

You do not need to examine her.

You have 10 minutes for this task (+ 2mins initial reading time).

Instructions for Assessor

Please read the instructions for the candidate and the role player.

Allow the candidate to conduct the consultation uninterrupted. If the candidate appears to be veering off course, gently prompt them showing the instruction sheet again.

Ascertain that the Candidate has:

- Assessed suitability of Nexplanon for this patient
- Explained to the patient the association between venous thromboembolism and Nexplanon use—no increase in risk
- Explained to the patient the drug interactions between Nexplanon and Lamotrigine—none as Lamotrigine is not an enzyme inducer
- Explained to the patient the association between obesity and Nexplanon use. Obesity is a UK MEC 1 with no restriction to use of Nexplanon
- Explained to the patient all the relevant points of Nexplanon use
- Excluded contraindications to the use of Implanon
- Identified the necessity for STI screening
- Sensitively addressed the importance of sexual health promotion

Record your clinical impression (Pass, Borderline, or Fail) for the candidate on each of the four domains.

Instructions for Role Player

You are Julie Smith, aged 24. You work part-time at a local supermarket as a shop assistant. You are 'on benefits' to support your two children aged six and three.

You have not had much luck with relationships recently and went through two 'split-ups' in the last year. You are seeking reliable contraception 'not associated with private areas'.

Your periods are regular and not heavy, although you would prefer it if they were less painful. You are certainly not keen on pregnancy anytime soon, however you would like to keep the option of childbearing open should 'you meet the right man'.

If specifically asked you admit to occasional vaginal bleeding after sexual intercourse and share the information that you take Lamotrigine for partial seizures. The seizures are well controlled and your last seizure was more than seven years ago. You have not had any problems in pregnancy from Lamotrigine use. You give the information that both your parents had venous thromboembolism and your granddad also had a clot in the lungs—pulmonary embolism.

You are overweight with a BMI of 38. You smoke and drink socially.

You do not consider yourself at risk of sexually transmitted infection, yet once pointed out to you that you may be at risk, you accept this and acknowledge the need for both STI screening and condom use for your own health.

You have had experience with almost all of the methods of contraception, but you were not satisfied with any. You blame the Depo-Provera injection for your weight gain. The coil gave you chronic pelvic pain. You could not remember to take the pills on time. Hence your wish for the implant. You also wish to use a method 'far removed from the genital area'.

Ideas: You are not expecting an internal examination. You are initially shocked when the Doctor suggests STI screening; however you soon accept it as necessary.

Concerns:

- Weight gain as you are already overweight
- Acne
- Libido
- Headaches
- Insertion process

You only reveal these concerns when specifically asked. When the candidate gives the information on these concerns anyway you should appear definitely pleased.

Expectations: You are expecting detailed information about the contraceptive implant. You are disappointed where the candidate only gives you sketchy information.

Assessment

Marking Scheme

Patient safety:

Pass	Borderline	Fail

Communication with patients and their relatives:

Pass	Borderline	Fail

Information gathering:

Pass	Borderline	Fail

Applied clinical knowledge:

Pass	Borderline	Fail

Notes for Marking

Patient safety

- Involves the patient in the decision making process, encouraging them to express their ideas and their preferences
- Addresses the importance of sexual health screening in the situation
- Sensitively addresses sexual health promotion—use of condoms
- Negotiates a mutually agreed acceptable plan
- Contraceptive precautions
- Non-judgemental approach to patient's lifestyle
- Open and honest about the side effects without being patronizing.
- Confidentiality of STI screening

Communication with the patients and their relatives

- Greets the patient and confirms patient identity
- Introduces themselves and their role in the health setting
- Explains the nature of the consultation
- Assesses the starting point for the patient
- Clear, organized information given in logical sequence
- Provides information in reasonable chunks
- Checks patient's understanding
- Uses clear language and avoids medical jargon
- Recognizes, acknowledges and validates patient concerns and feelings and is empathetic

Information gathering

- Obtains a focussed history relevant to the task
- Obtains patients views, expectations, and concerns

Applied clinical knowledge

- Demonstrates sound and comprehensive evidence-based clinical knowledge and familiarity with the contraceptive implant
- Assesses the suitability by excluding contraindications to use based on UK MEC
- Counsels the patient with the relevant information, that is factually correct on:
- Indications
- Duration of use
- Mechanism of action—primary and secondary
- Health benefits viz dysmenorrhoea
- Risks of problematic bleeding that does not change with time
- Failure rate of 0.05%
- Side effects of acne, headache, weight gain, mood changes and libido
- No increase in risk of venous thromboembolism/myocardial infarction or decreased bone mineral density
- Timing of insertion

- Drug interactions with Lamotrigine
- Obesity association
- Insertion techniques under local anaesthesia
- Follow up not routinely required unless the patient wishes
- Follow up for side effects if patient wishes
- Symptoms to watch out for viz: pregnancy, cannot feel the Nexplanon or changes to the size and shape of the Nexplanon, or skin changes
- Rapid return to fertility after removal
- Appropriate non-verbal behaviour with eye contact, posture, position, facial expression, use of voice, pace, and tone

Notes for Candidate

This is a counselling station that assesses:

- Your knowledge of the contraceptive implant.
- Your communication skills and history taking.
- The ability to sensitively address sexually transmitted infection screening.
- The ability to maintain a non-judgemental approach.
- Identification of the wider issues of sexual health promotion.

Further reading

Contraceptive Choices for Young People Clinical Effectiveness Unit, Faculty of Sexual & Reproductive Health Care; March 2010. https://www.fsrh.org/documents/ … /cec-ceu-guidance-young-people-mar-2010.pdf

Task 3 **Termination of pregnancy**

Instructions for Candidate

This task assesses the following clinical skills:

- Patient safety
- Communication with patients
- Information gathering
- Applied clinical knowledge

You are an ST5 doctor, on call for Gynaecology. You have accepted a 38 year old patient, Jeanette Simpson, from A&E who has been bleeding heavily after a termination of pregnancy two weeks ago. She is haemodynamically stable and is sitting in the treatment room of the Gynaecology Ward, waiting for a bed. Her observations are normal. Please take a brief history and formulate a list of differential diagnoses.

After taking the history you will be asked to give a brief summary of the relevant points and list your differential diagnoses to the assessor.

You will then be given the examination findings by the assessor and asked to make a definitive diagnosis and management plan. You will then explain these to the patient.

You have 10 minutes for this task (+ 2mins initial reading time).

Instruction for Assessor

Please show instructions to candidate and actor.

Allow the candidate to conduct the interview undisturbed unless they are straying off the track of the question (in which case show them their instructions again).

This patient has retained products of conception after medical TOP. The history should include:

- Gestation at termination
- Scan (TAS/TVS) prior to procedure
- Confirmation that it was a medical procedure with all prescribed tablets taken correctly
- What happened after the tablets were taken –pain, bleeding, clots, passage of obvious gestation sac
- Bleeding and pain since then—timing, duration, severity
- Presence/absence of pregnancy symptoms
- Temperature, fever or rigors
- Offensive vaginal discharge
- Any unilateral pain, faintness, or shoulder tip pain.
- PMH specifically past O&G history, eliciting post-partum haemorrhage and heavy bleed following miscarriage
- Bleeding tendency
- Smear history

Differential diagnosis:

- Incomplete termination of pregnancy with retained products of conception (RPOC)
- Endometritis
- Failed termination of pregnancy (ongoing pregnancy)
- Ectopic pregnancy

Once the candidate has taken a relevant history and presented it to you with a list of differential diagnosis, provide the candidate with the following information:

- Observations—pulse 80 bpm BP 120/75 mmHg T 37.5°C BMI 40
- Abdominal examination—suprapubic tenderness, no guarding or rebound
- Speculum examination—parous os with some fresh red blood in the vaginal vault
- Bimanual examination—generally tender, uterus 6/40 size (limited due to BMI), no cervical excitation, adnexae NAD
- Transvaginal scan—products of conception seen in the uterine cavity measuring 33 x 43 x 27mm. Ovaries NAD. No free fluid. The patient found the scan uncomfortable but no specific probe tenderness.
- Urinary pregnancy test positive
- Serum β HCG 600mIU/ml
- Haemoglobin 103g/L

Now ask the candidate to make a definitive diagnosis and explain both the diagnosis and the most appropriate management plan to Jeanette

There are some marks on the process mark sheet for the actor to assign at the end of the station.

Record your overall clinical impression of the candidate for each domain (i.e. should this performance be pass, borderline, or a fail).

Instructions for Role Player

You are Jeanette Simpson, a 38-year-old mother of two teenage children. Both children were vaginal deliveries and each weighed 10 + lbs but the first one was complicated by a postpartum haemorrhage. You had two units of blood transfused before being discharged. You have also had a complete miscarriage five years ago not requiring any hospital treatment except scans. You were anaemic after the miscarriage and this was treated with iron.

Two weeks ago you had a termination of pregnancy (TOP). You conceived whilst taking the mini pill (or 'progesterone only pill') and requested termination because your family is complete. You were six weeks pregnant and opted for a home medical procedure, taking two doses of tablets at the clinic six hours apart, before going home to complete the abortion process. You experienced cramps and heavy bleeding with large clots similar to when you had the miscarriage and presumed that you had passed the pregnancy.

Everything settled down but a week later you started to experience intermittent gushes of blood. This has been going on for a further week and happens roughly every other day. Today you have passed a fist sized clot and more blood in A&E. The bleeding seems to have stopped now.

You were instructed to check a pregnancy test four weeks after the procedure but you have actually done one today because you are worried and the test is positive.

If you are specifically asked:

- You had an abdominal 'tummy' scan before the termination
- You experience generalized, central cramping pains prior to the 'gushes' of blood but nothing in between episodes. A gush typically soaks through two or three maternity pads over an hour and then tails off
- You *did not* see an obvious gestation sac (pregnancy sac) when you were bleeding after the tablets
- You *do not* have ongoing pregnancy symptoms (sore breasts, nausea)
- You *do not* have a temperature or feel feverish—just tired and worn out

- You *have not* had an offensive vaginal discharge associated with the bleeding
- Your periods have always been heavy
- You are overweight but in good health with no medications except the mini pill and no allergies. Your smears are normal and up to date
- You are going to see your GP about having a Mirena 'hormone coil' fitted for ongoing contraception and to help your heavy periods
- There are no serious illnesses in the family

Temperament: You were upset about having to have a termination but you and your husband were sure of the decision. The ongoing bleeding is making you feel much worse though as you thought it would be over and done with by now.

Ideas: Your main fear is that you are still pregnant in spite of the tablets.

Concerns: You are hoping for a definitive treatment such as surgical management.

Expectations: When the doctor has the scan result you want the following explained clearly to you:

- It is not an ongoing pregnancy but there seems to be some pregnancy tissue and blood clot in the womb
- Because the bleeding is continuing, you will need to go to theatre for an Evacuation of Retained Products of Conception so that the tissue can be removed from the womb using suction, whilst you are asleep
- Risks and benefits of the procedure
- When you can go home

Assessment

Marking Scheme

Patient safety:

Pass	Borderline	Fail

Communication with patients and their relatives:

Pass	Borderline	Fail

Information gathering:

Pass	Borderline	Fail

Applied clinical knowledge:

Pass	Borderline	Fail

Notes for Marking

Patient safety

- Assesses patient's main concerns and ideas
- Explains diagnosis clearly
- Makes appropriate plan—surgical management in view of ongoing, intermittent, heavy blood loss
- Discusses risks and benefits
- Checks future contraception

Communication with patients and their relatives

- Greets, introduces self and role, checks patient's name
- Consent to proceed and explains nature of interview
- Assesses patient's starting point (what the patient wants to know) and sets the agenda
- Clear organized explanation in logical sequence
- Chunks: i.e. provides information in reasonable chunks
- Checks patient's understanding.
- Language (easily understood, avoids or explains jargon)
- Uses visual aids appropriately e.g. diagrams or uses analogies to aid explanation

Information gathering

- Obtains a focussed history relevant to the task
- Obtains patients views, expectations, and concerns

Applied clinical knowledge

- Demonstrates a sound and comprehensive evidence-based clinical knowledge
- Elicits all relevant history
- Formulates logical and likely differential diagnoses, considers ectopic pregnancy
- Uses examination and investigation findings to refine diagnosis

Notes for Candidate

History taking

- The information you are given clearly indicates that this woman is haemodynamically stable. This is not an acutely life-threatening scenario
- UK law allows conscientious objection to abortion to be exercised in relation to providing the abortion procedure itself but not to treating complications
- Doctors with conscientious objection to abortion should be familiar with the theory of medical and surgical procedures and their local service provision to enable them to treat complications effectively
- Undiagnosed ectopic pregnancy must be excluded
- It is important to understand the difference between a *failed* termination (with an ongoing, viable pregnancy) and an *incomplete* termination (with retained products of conception) and ensure accurate documentation
- Compliance with treatment– ambivalence and/or fear may prevent women from completing treatment, increasing the risk of ongoing pregnancy
- Ensure that a contraceptive plan is in place

Diagnosis and management

- Transvaginal scan helps to exclude ongoing or ectopic pregnancy
- In this case the scan findings are clear and compatible with the clinical picture. In other cases, serial β HCGs may be required
- The positive pregnancy test reflects the presence of retained tissue rather than a viable pregnancy

- Definitive surgical treatment is the correct management in this case on clinical grounds—significant symptoms not improving, previous obstetric haemorrhage
- Contraception should be started immediately after TOP

Further reading

Best practice in comprehensive post abortion care. Best Practice Paper No 3. March 2016. Leading Safe Choices. www.rcog.org.uk

Contraception After Pregnancy Jan 2017. CEU Clinical Guidance. www.fsrh.org.uk

Task 4 **Sexually Transmitted Infections and HIV**

Instructions for Candidate

This task assesses the following clinical skills:

- Patient safety
- Communication with patients and their relatives
- Information gathering
- Applied clinical knowledge

You are an ST4 doctor working in an obstetric clinic. Your consultant has just been called to theatre and so the midwife has asked you to see Lucy Hardwick, a 22-year-old, 14 weeks pregnant lady who has just been told her antenatal screening test is positive for HIV. No high risk for HIV was identified prior to the screening test. Please take a history and explain the diagnosis and outline the management plan. You do not need to examine her. Once you have completed the consultation you will be asked to give a brief summary of the relevant points in the history to the assessor.

You will be given surrogate marker test results and asked some questions by the assessor.

You have 10 minutes for this task (+ 2mins initial reading time).

Instruction for Assessor

Please read instructions to candidate and actor.

Allow the candidate to conduct the interview undisturbed unless they are straying off the track of the question (in which case you can show them their instructions again).

The candidate should allow the actor to ask any pressing questions not answered by the midwife, prior to taking a history. The candidate may have to outline the natural history and treatment of HIV along with its transmission early in the consultation. The candidate may have to ask permission to pause the role player's questions and take a medical and sexual history in order to inform answers.

The history should cover:

- Current health
- Past illnesses
- Systems review (cough, shortness of breath, fever, sweats, appetite, weight, diarrhoea, headache, skin problems)
- Menstrual and cervical cytology history
- Obstetric history including previous antenatal screening
- Sexual history (partner/s since last HIV negative test, contraception, barrier methods)
- Blood borne virus history (injecting drug use, partner/s injecting drugs/ bisexual/from high risk country, commercial sex work)
- If history of thrush/TV elicited, details of discharge, dysuria and post coital bleeding should be taken
- Family history, social history
- Current drug history

Once the candidate has taken a relevant history and presented to you, provide the candidate with the following information:

CD4 count 690/mm3
Viral load 11,334 HIV RNA copies/ml

Now ask the candidate to explain the likely route of acquisition of HIV and the management plan to Lucy. The candidate should have identified that Harry was at risk of HIV acquisition if Lucy seroconverted to HIV positive late in her first pregnancy. Testing for Harry should be discussed and arranged.

There are some marks on the process mark sheet for the actor to assign at the end of the station.

Record your overall clinical impression of the candidate for each domain (e.g. should this performance be pass, borderline, or a fail).

Instructions for Role Player

You are Lucy Hardwick, aged 22 years. You are a full-time mum for Harry aged 18 months. You have been with your partner John for three years. John is a 26-year-old mechanic who moved to your area from London three years ago. His family are from Zimbabwe and he left Zimbabwe, aged 20 years, to study in the UK. John works away every other week, but you feel well supported by your mum who lives nearby and likes spending lots of time with you and Harry. You have had no other pregnancies and have occasionally used condoms. You knew you had an HIV screening test done recently but were not worried about the result as you remember it had been negative when you were tested early in your first pregnancy with Harry two years ago. You had told the midwife that John was from Africa when you were pregnant with Harry, but as the midwife made no comment and the test was negative you didn't think it important to mention this again earlier in this pregnancy,

If you are specifically asked:

- In the past you have never had any major illnesses, but do suffer from recurrent 'thrush'. This causes lots of vaginal discharge, smell and sometimes itching
- You have not lost any weight
- You have no other symptoms (shortness of breath, skin problems, fever, sweats, diarrhoea etc.)
- Your cervical smears have shown wart virus infection and TV
- You have never injected drugs
- You have had no new sexual partners since your previous antenatal HIV negative test two years ago

Temperament: You think you are sensible and generally 'sorted', but emotional when tired. Harry hasn't been sleeping well recently and he's in the waiting room with your mum. You are very anxious as you were called back to clinic unexpectedly and you thought something must be wrong with the baby.

Ideas: Initially you can't believe this test is right as you were negative when last tested. You are confused as to how this could have happened.

Concerns: You are worried your children might get AIDS and you will get ill and not be able to look after them. You are worried about how to tell your partner.

Expectations: You want the doctor to explain the following:

- How this could have happened
- What you can do to protect the children
- If there are any treatments, you can have which won't damage the baby
- How long have you have got to live

Assessment

Marking Scheme

Patient safety:

Pass Borderline Fail

Communication with patients and their relatives:

Pass Borderline Fail

Information gathering:

Pass Borderline Fail

Applied clinical knowledge:

Pass Borderline Fail

Notes for Marking

Patient safety

- Assesses the patient's main concerns and ideas
- Explains HIV transmissions may occur years into a monogamous relationship and that vertical transmission unlikely with appropriate intervention. Facilitates testing of partner and first child. Discusses that HIV medication taken is unlikely to cause foetal abnormality or toxicity.
- Involves patient in the process (e.g. encouraging them to express their ideas, or preferences
- Negotiates a mutually agreed acceptable, safe, plan
- Open and honest about antiretroviral use and possible complications
- Advises on the provision of written information to consider prior to medication
- Negotiates a plan for testing child and baby in a timely fashion taking into account the patient's concerns. Being honest about small risk to baby if intervention acceptable, and of risk to toddler plus likely infection in partner

Communication with patients and their relatives

- Greets, introduces self and role, checks patient's name
- Consent to proceed and explains nature of interview
- Assesses patient's starting point (what the patient wants to know) and sets the agenda
- Clear organized explanation in logical sequence
- Chunks: e.g. provides information in reasonable chunks
- Checks patient's understanding
- Language (easily understood, avoids or explains jargon)
- Uses visual aids appropriately e.g. diagrams or uses analogies to aid explanation
- Presents a clear and succinct history to the assessor

Information gathering

The history should cover:

- Current health
- Past illnesses

- Systems review (cough, shortness of breath, fever, sweats, appetite, weight, diarrhoea, headache, skin problems)
- Menstrual and cervical cytology history
- Obstetric history including previous antenatal screening
- Sexual history (partner/s since last HIV negative test, contraception, barrier methods)
- Blood borne virus history (injecting drug use, partner/s injecting drugs/ bisexual/from high risk country, commercial sex work)
- If history of thrush/TV elicited, details of discharge, dysuria and post coital bleeding should be taken
- Family history, social history
- Current drug history

Applied clinical knowledge

Demonstrates a sound and comprehensive evidence-based clinical knowledge—e.g. is able to confirm that with such a CD4 count and viral load the patient is not likely to have any HIV related illnesses, but will need treatment to prevent vertical transmission to the baby. The candidate should be aware that with appropriate use of antiretroviral therapy her HIV infection is not likely to adversely affect her life expectancy. Investigation for other sexually transmitted infections should be arranged for a later date in view of the vaginal discharge and history of trichomonas vaginalis.

Further reading

Familiarize yourself with the BASHH HIV guidelines. https://www.bashh.org/guidelines

Task 5 **Vaginismus**

Instructions for Candidate

This task assesses the following clinical skills:

- Patient safety
- Communication with patients
- Information gathering
- Applied clinical knowledge

You are an ST4 doctor working in a gynaecology clinic with your consultant. Your consultant has asked you to take relevant history from Rachel Barford who is a 28-year-old who has been referred by her GP for dyspareunia. She is a fit and healthy mother of one with a past medical history of mild asthma and an eating disorder in her late teens. Please take an appropriate history using six minutes of your allocated time. You will then be asked to give a brief summary of the relevant points in the history to the assessor

You will be given the examination findings and asked some questions by the assessor.

You have 10 minutes for this task (+ 2mins initial reading time).

Instruction for Assessor

Please read instructions to candidate and actor.

Allow the candidate to conduct the interview undisturbed unless they are straying off the track of the question (in which case you can show them their instructions again).

This patient has dyspareunia caused by vaginismus. The history of presenting complaint should cover:

- The onset, duration and nature of the pain
- Establishing that it is superficial not deep dyspareunia
- Any intermenstrual or post coital bleeding
- Smear history
- Contraception
- PMH, DH and allergies
- Family history and social history

Once the candidate has taken a relevant history and presented it to you, provide the candidate with the following information:

- Abdominal examination—unremarkable
- Speculum examination—some resistance to full insertion but possible. Not possible to open speculum due to muscle tension and discomfort. No evidence of scar tissue or abnormally restricted or scarred introitus
- Bimanual examination—muscle tension at vaginal entrance, gradually able to overcome. Uterus small, anteverted, non-tender, adnexae NAD. Patient reports severe burning pain at withdrawal of fingers

Now ask the candidate what they think the working diagnosis is and to explain it to Rachel. Also, what can be done about it?

There are some marks on the process mark sheet for the actor to assign at the end of the station.

Record your overall clinical impression of the candidate for each domain (e.g. should this performance be pass, borderline, or a fail).

Instructions for Role Player

You are Rachel Barford, aged 28. You are married to James, 35 and you have been together for six years. You met whilst both working for a PR agency and have been married for four years. At the beginning of your relationship sex was fine but since the birth of your daughter, Hollie, aged two years, it has been so painful that you have only had sex a couple of times since she was born. The pain is all around the entrance to the vagina and feels almost like a 'block'. You experience a burning pain if penetration does occur and this lasts for a day after sex. You do not have any pelvic pain.

The delivery was a horrendous experience and came as a complete shock because you assumed that you would cope well with it. You were fit, healthy and going to the gym right up to the end. The pregnancy was fine and you planned to return to work full time. You were induced because you were overdue and had a spontaneous vaginal delivery 2 days after the induction began. The induction process was slow, and for the first day after the pessaries you were sure you were having labour contractions as the pain was so bad but the midwives kept saying you weren't in established labour. The vaginal examinations to check on progress after the pessaries were the most painful thing you have ever experienced in your life. When you were ready to go to the labour ward this was delayed for a day as there was no room available. You had not slept since admission and very soon found yourself with a drip and epidural—neither of which you had envisaged yourself having. You pushed for two hours and finally delivered after an episiotomy (another thing you had not wanted) because the baby was getting tired. You have a clear memory of lying with your legs up, with several people in the room, most of whom seemed to be peering between your legs at one point or other and the doctor doing the repair having to ask yet another person to come and look.

After you went home you were terrified in case the episiotomy broke down or didn't heal well and waited for six months before trying to have sex again. You were not really interested but felt that you should for your husband's sake. He has never pressurized you for sex. It was so painful that you had to stop and penetration was impossible due to pain and the feeling of a 'block'.

When your smear was due it was so painful that it had to be abandoned and you told the nurse about pain with sex and so were referred to gynaecology.

If you are specifically asked:

- In the past you have had an eating disorder in your teens during which you restricted your calorie intake and exercised excessively. You had some counselling sessions which helped you regain a healthier balance
- You have a blue inhaler for asthma and hardly ever use it
- The pain during sex is like a brick wall at the entrance to the vagina with the pain felt just inside the entrance. It starts to feel like a burning pain if penetration succeeds and lasts for about a day afterwards
- Sex was fine before the birth
- There is no bleeding after sex
- Your first smear age 25 did not hurt and the results were normal
- You have not used tampons since the birth because you do not bleed with the pill you are on but used to get on okay with them
- You are taking the mini pill for contraception, and you are very particular about taking it as you don't want to get pregnant again
- There is no family history of note

Temperament: You like to be prepared and in control in your life but the dyspareunia makes you feel helpless and frustrated.

Ideas: You wonder if perhaps there is some scar tissue from the episiotomy or whether the repair was made too tight. You are hoping that an operation will be suggested which will cure the problem

Concerns: You are worried that this has gone on so long. Repeated reassurances that everything is physically alright are simply frustrating because there is obviously some kind of problem.

Expectations: You want the doctor to:

- Take you seriously even though this is an awkward problem
- Listen carefully to your concerns (that there is something physically wrong even though the GP and practice nurse have said there is not)
- Believe that the pain is real not just 'in your head'
- Explain what vaginismus is
- Explain how vaginismus can be related to or triggered by emotionally and physically painful events
- What can be done about it?

Assessment

Marking Scheme

Patient safety:
Pass Borderline Fail

Communication with patients and their relatives:
Pass Borderline Fail

Information gathering:
Pass Borderline Fail

Applied clinical knowledge:
Pass Borderline Fail

Notes for Marking

Patient safety

- 'Permission' is given to the patient by the doctor's attitude to discuss sex and to discuss feelings about delivery
- Open and honest about diagnosis—is careful to be clear that surgery is not indicated
- Avoid giving the impression that it is all in the patient's head—it is a real problem, with real physical symptoms but has emotional and psychological triggers

Information gathering

- Obtains a relevant sexual history
- Obtains patients views, expectations, and concerns

Communication with patients and their relatives

- Greets, introduces self and role, checks patient's name
- Consent to proceed and explains nature of interview
- Asks questions about sex in a clear, open, unembarrassed way which enables the patient to speak frankly
- Allows patient to give information uninterrupted
- Is able to allow patient to be upset and acknowledges tears or anger or frustration

- Language (easily understood, avoids or explains jargon)
- Presents a clear and succinct history to the assessor
- Communicate the diagnosis of vaginismus clearly
- Explains the connection between physically and emotionally painful events which might trigger a physical response.
- Addresses the patient's main concerns and ideas—explain that the vagina is anatomically normal (i.e. no scar tissue) but that pain is real and coming from muscle tension
- Explains that an operation would create scar tissue and not help
- Options for management include psychosexual counselling, pelvic floor physiotherapy and/or use of vaginal trainers
- Involves patient in the process (e.g. encouraging them to express their ideas, or preferences)
- Uses visual aids appropriately e.g. diagrams or uses analogies to aid explanation
- Negotiates a mutually agreed acceptable, safe, plan

Applied clinical knowledge

- Demonstrates a sound and comprehensive evidence-based clinical knowledge—e.g. takes relevant history to exclude physical causes, takes sexual history and correctly relates problems to birth of baby, enquires about other penetrative causes of pain (tampon use) as well as smears and sex
- Makes correct diagnosis when given examination findings

Notes for Candidate

This patient has been traumatized by what may seem to an obstetrician to be a relatively straightforward delivery resulting in a healthy baby and a healthy mother. It is vital to be able to adopt the patient's perspective which is one of unexpectedly severe pain and a loss of control over events in an individual who is used to being in control. The doctor is more likely to be able to establish rapport if he/she can avoid interpreting this patient's history as an implicit criticism of medical care as this may lead to an unhelpfully defensive response from the doctor.

Further reading

Crowley T, Goldmeier D, Hiller J. Diagnosing and managing vaginismus, Clinical Review. *BMJ*, 2009. 338: b2284 doi: 10.1136/bmj.b2284. https://www.bashh.org/documents/2429.pdf

Helping People with Sexual Problems: a practical approach for clinicians. Peter Trigwell.

Chapter 17 Early Pregnancy Care

Task 1 Ectopic Pregnancy

Instructions for Candidate

This task assesses the following clinical skills:

- Patient safety
- Communication with patients and their relatives
- Information gathering
- Applied clinical knowledge

You are an ST4 doctor covering Early Pregnancy Assessment Unit (EPAU). You have been asked to see 24-year-old Jaz Pringle in her third pregnancy.

Her LMP was six weeks ago and has presented with left iliac fossa pain and light vaginal bleeding.

Your task is:

- To take a focussed history
- Organize the necessary investigations
- Discuss the results and diagnosis with Jaz
- Agree a management plan

You have 10 minutes for this task (+ 2mins initial reading time).

Instruction for Assessor

This is a communication skills clinical assessment task that tests the candidate's skills to take a focussed history, interpret and explain results and agree to a management plan having discussed the options.

If they ask for the urine pregnancy test, tell them it is positive.

If they arrange an ultrasound, provide them with the following result.

'An empty uterus and a 2.3cm left sided adnexal mass with well-defined gestational sac medial to the left ovary with minimal fluid in pouch of Douglas. Right ovary appeared normal. Findings are highly suggestive of left sided tubal pregnancy'.

If they organize beta HCG, tell them the nurse had sent it and the result is back and it is 2900IU/ml.

Record your overall clinical impression of the candidate for each domain (e.g. should this performance be pass, borderline, or a fail).

Instructions for Role Player

You are Ms. Jaz Pringle, a 24-year-old housewife who lives with her partner of four years. You have one child delivered by caesarean section for breech (bottom first) presentation three years ago. You had developed infection post caesarean section and were very unwell. You had needed admission to the hospital for 10 days and needed IV antibiotics.

This was followed by an ectopic pregnancy 18 months ago whereby you ended up having key hole surgery and removal of your right fallopian tube with ectopic pregnancy. While you have not been actively trying for another pregnancy, you and your partner are happy with the thought of another pregnancy.

However, you attended hospital due to some discomfort on the left side of the tummy and some vaginal bleeding on and off for two days.

You are otherwise fit and well with no allergies.

The candidate should arrange a urine pregnancy test, which will be positive. They should then organize a scan in the EPAU. The scan will suggest an ectopic pregnancy in your right tube.

You are now extremely upset and anxious after the scan at the thought of possibly losing the only remaining tube and being rendered infertile. You want to know all possible options and would like to save the only fallopian tube if possible.

You want the doctor to:

- Show empathy
- Explain the diagnosis of tubal ectopic pregnancy based on scan and blood test results
- Why you are having repeated ectopic pregnancies
- Possible options for management-surgical, medical and conservative
- Benefits and risks in details on medical management as you prefer this option (success rate, possibility of repeat treatment, possibility of surgery, side-effects of medication, do's and don't's)
- Address your concerns about future fertility in the context of having only one fallopian tube
- Help reach a shared decision for management

Assessment

Marking Scheme

Patient safety:

Pass Borderline Fail

Communication with patients and their relatives:

Pass Borderline Fail

Information gathering:

Pass Borderline Fail

Applied clinical knowledge:

Pass Borderline Fail

Notes for Marking

Patient safety

- Assesses the patient's main concerns
- Involves patient in the process (e.g. encouraging them to express their ideas, or preferences)
- Negotiates a mutually agreed acceptable, safe, plan
- Open and honest about the result without being patronizing
- Open and honest about the risks

Communication with patients and their relatives

- Greets patient and obtains patient's name
- Introduces self, role

- Explains nature of interview (reason for coming to talk to patient)
- Assesses starting point: what patient understands already/is feeling
- Gives clear signposting that important information is to follow
- Uses patient's response to guide next steps
- Discovers what other information would help the patient, attempts to address patient's information needs
- Gives explanation in an organized manner (signposting/summarising)
- Uses clear language, avoids jargon and confusing language
- Picks up and responds to patient's non-verbal cues
- Allows patient time to react (use of silence, allows for shut-down)
- Recognizes, acknowledges and validates patient's concerns and feelings (e.g. uses empathy)
- Appropriate non-verbal behaviour e.g. eye contact, posture and position, movement, facial expression, use of voice (pace, tone)
- Provides support: e.g. concern, understanding, willingness to help
- Avoids platitudes or false re-assurance

Information gathering

- Obtains a focussed and relevant history
- Obtains patient's views, expectations, and concerns

Applied clinical knowledge

- Organizes urine pregnancy test, ultrasound and serum beta HCG
- Identifies postpartum infection, previous caesarean sections, and previous laparoscopic surgery as the risk factors for repeat ectopic pregnancy
- Can interpret the ultrasound scan and explain to Jaz the diagnosis of left ectopic pregnancy
- Discusses option of Methotrexate and laparoscopic left salpingectomy
- Discusses the limitations and risks of methotrexate treatment, including possibility of a repeat ectopic pregnancy
- Discusses implications of left salpingectomy, mainly infertility

Further reading

Diagnosis and Management of Ectopic Pregnancy (Green-top Guideline No. 21; Joint with the Association of Early Pregnancy Units) 04/11/2016. https://www.rcog.org.uk/en/guidelines-research-services/guidelines/gtg21/

Ectopic pregnancy and miscarriage: diagnosis and initial management, Clinical guideline [CG154 Published date: December 2012]. https://www.nice.org.uk/guidance/cg154

Task 2 **Early pregnancy problem with IUCD**

Instructions for Candidate

This task assesses the following clinical skills:

- Patient safety
- Communication with patients and their relatives
- Information gathering
- Applied clinical knowledge

You are an ST3 doctor covering Early Pregnancy Assessment Unit. Marjorie Brand a 26-year-old mother of two has presented with persistent vaginal spotting for a week. She has a copper IUCD in place and her periods have been very irregular recently. Her pregnancy test is positive and an ultrasound scan has been organized at the Early Pregnancy Unit by her GP.

You are tasked with:

- Taking a focussed history
- Explain the ultrasound scan findings
- Discuss possible management options
- Address patient's concerns if any

You have 10 minutes for this task (+ 2mins initial reading time).

Instructions for Assessor

This is a clinical knowledge and communication skills station testing the candidate's ability to take relevant history, communicate results of ultrasound scan, and provide relevant clinical information on the topic to the patient to help agree on a management plan.

If the candidate, ask for the ultrasound scan the results are as follows:

- Single intrauterine pregnancy with CRL corresponding to ten weeks' pregnancy. Foetal heart and foetal movements noted. IUCD noted low in uterine cavity. No evidence of any hematomas and no adnexal masses
- Record your overall clinical impression of the candidate for each domain (e.g. should this performance be pass, borderline or a fail)

Instructions for Role Player

You are Miss Marjorie Brand, a 26-year-old school teacher. You live with your partner and two children, aged three and one. Both your pregnancies were uncomplicated resulting in normal vaginal delivery. You now have a copper IUD in place for contraception inserted at a local family planning clinic eight months ago. Your periods have become quite irregular since coil insertion and in recent months, periods have been lighter than normal with persistent spotting for a week now.

Apart from history of appendicectomy at the age of 18 and mild bronchial asthma, for which you take Ventolin inhaler, you are fit and well.

Your pregnancy test was positive at your doctor's surgery. Your doctor has referred you to the early pregnancy assessment unit for an ultrasound scan. The scan confirms a viable intrauterine pregnancy of ten weeks' gestation (ten weeks' size pregnancy with heart beat noted on scan) along with a copper coil in the womb.

You are obviously a bit upset at the thought of this unplanned pregnancy and concerned about the implications of pregnancy with the coil in the womb.

If asked by the doctor after consideration of the information provided, you will agree an internal examination and removal of the coil.

You would like the doctor to:

- Explain the scan findings
- Be empathetic explaining the diagnosis of this unplanned but viable intrauterine pregnancy
- Address your thoughts on this pregnancy (if asked, you would like to keep this pregnancy)
- Explain the need for undertaking a speculum/internal examination
- Address your questions: Should the coil be removed now or removed later or left alone?
- Provide you with information to make decision

Assessment

Marking Scheme

Patient safety:

Pass Borderline Fail

Communication with patients and their relatives:

Pass Borderline Fail

Information gathering:

Pass Borderline Fail

Applied clinical knowledge:

Pass Borderline Fail

Notes for Marking

Patient safety

- Assesses patient's main concerns
- Able to help patient reach an informed decision about removing or leaving the coil based on available evidence
- Open and honest without patronizing
- If unable to answer any queries correctly, offers to seek help from consultant/senior medical staff.

Communication with patients and their relatives

- Greets the patient, checks patient identity
- Introduces self and job role
- Understands patient's feelings about being told she is pregnant despite having a coil in the womb for contraception
- Shows empathy
- Picks up and reacts to patient's non-verbal clues
- Explains in a logical manner in lay terms avoiding jargon

- Allows time for patient to understand and ask questions
- Provision of support/written information

Information gathering

- Obtains a focussed and relevant history
- Obtains patient's views, expectations, and concerns

Applied clinical knowledge

- Ability to interpret the scan results and explain to patient
- Ability to acknowledge patient's views on the issue
- Ability to reassure the patient and answer patient's queries about removing the coil now or later or leaving the coil in place for rest of the pregnancy
- Reassure the patient and help reach the best decision which in this situation would be to remove the coil if threads are seen on examination, the chances of which are good especially with the scan also reporting the coil to be placed low in the womb cavity and patient being only ten weeks pregnant

Notes for Candidate

As per NICE guidance on long term reversible contraception, 2005—if coil threads are visible or easily retrievable on speculum examination, then it should be removed before 12 weeks' of gestation. Risks of miscarriage can be as high as 50–60% with coil left *in situ* compared to 10–15% background risk of miscarriage. Removal of coil although associated with a small risk of miscarriage, this risk is much lower and overall risks of miscarriage, infection and preterm delivery are lower if coil is removed before 12 week's pregnancy.

Further reading

IUD removal in pregnancy (query bank), RCOG. www.rcog.org.uk/en/guidelines-research-services/guidelines/iud-removal-in-pregnancy---query-bank/

Task 3 **Hyperemesis**

Instructions for Candidate

This task assesses the following clinical skills:

- Patient safety
- Communication with colleagues
- Applied clinical knowledge

Mrs Daniela Koszuk has been admitted to Gynae emergencies with multiple episodes of vomiting over the last 24 hours. She hasn't passed urine since last night and appears dry. On enquiry her last period was nine weeks ago and she had a positive pregnancy test four weeks ago. She has been suffering from nausea and vomiting for the last three weeks but recently it has been intractable and she's not able to keep anything down. As the on call registrar your task is:

- Request appropriate investigations
- Interpret data
- Discuss management options with the assessor

You have 10 minutes for this task (+ 2mins initial reading time).

Instructions for Assessor

This clinical assessment task is to assess the skills of the candidate to organize appropriate investigations to reach a diagnosis and discuss the management options in a case with Hyperemesis and possible Hydatidiform Mole.

Ask them what investigations they would organize.

They are expected to organize FBC, Us and Es, LFTs, TFTs, urinalysis, MSU, and transvaginal scan.

Show them the results of the investigations as they request them (Fig. 17.1, Fig. 17.2, and Table 17.1).

Results sheet A (Figure 17.1)

Date xx/xx/xxxx

Daniela Koszuk

Date of Birth: dd/mm/yy

Hospital no: xyx

Result sheet B

Ask them to comment on the results

Ask them the management of hyperemesis

What do they think is the likely cause of hyperemesis based on the scan findings?

Discuss the management of Hydatidiform Mole with you.

Table 17.1 Results

		Normal value
Hb:	129g/L	
Hct:	0.470	
WBC	12x10^9/L	
CRP	5	
TSH	0.52mu/L	0.35–3.50
FT$_3$:	4.3pmol/L	3.8–6.0
Free Thyroxine:	12pmol/L	8–21
Na	14 mmol/L	134–145
K	5.0mmol/L	3.6–5.0
Urea	4.3mmol/L	1.7–7.1
Creatinine	60umol/L	49–90
eGFR	>90	mL/min/1.73m^2
Total Bilirubin	10umol/L	0–22
Total Protein	67g/L	63–82
Albumin	40g/L	35–50
Globulin	27g/L	21–35
Alk. Phosph	52U/L	38–126
ALT	5 U/L	0–50
Urinalysis:	Ketones 3 +	

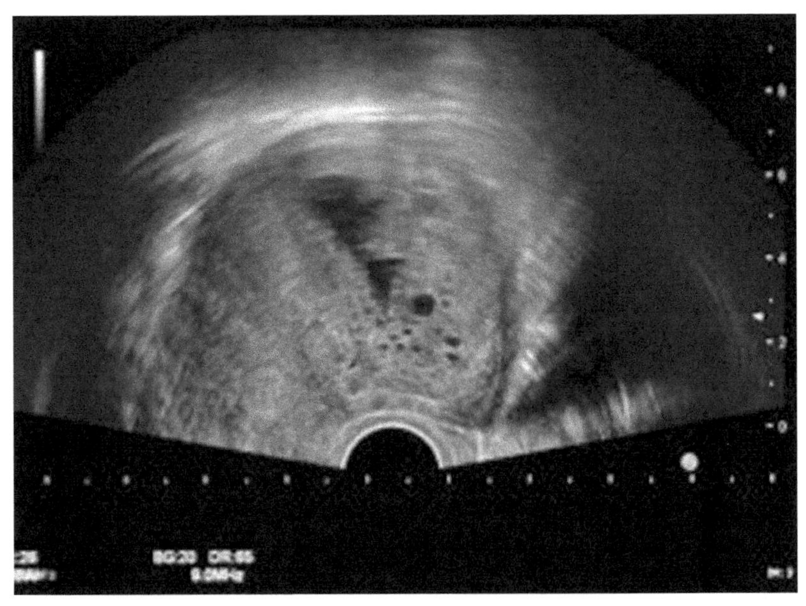

Fig. 17.1 Transvaginal ultrasound

Assessment

Marking Scheme		
Patient safety:		
Pass	Borderline	Fail
Communication with colleagues:		
Pass	Borderline	Fail
Information gathering:		
Pass	Borderline	Fail
Applied clinical knowledge:		
Pass	Borderline	Fail

Notes for Marking

Patient safety

- Confirms patient details on all investigations
- Discusses options and the pros and cons of each
- Quotes the most up to date guidelines for management

Communication with colleagues

- Clear and concise

Applied clinical knowledge

- Demonstrates a sound and comprehensive evidence-based clinical knowledge
- Requests appropriate investigations and interprets them accurately
- Can interpret scan findings
- Makes a provisional diagnosis and discusses differential diagnosis
- Discusses the management of hyperemesis and molar pregnancy based on up-to-date guidelines
- Discusses the importance of histological examination of the products of conception in diagnosis of molar pregnancy
- Suggests referral to the relevant trophoblastic screening centre
- Understands the importance of contraception until follow-up is complete (suggests barrier)

Notes for Candidate

Request for investigations including FBC, Us & Es, LFTs, TFTs, urinalysis, MSU, and transvaginal scan.

Patient safety and quality

Check patient details to confirm investigations of the right patient.

Interpretation of investigations

Comment on raised haematocrit suggestive of dehydration.

- CRP and WCC unlikely to be suggestive of infection
- Comment on normal TFTs

- Slightly raised ALT could be a cause as well as an effect of hyperemesis
- 3 + ketones on urine dip suggestive of significant dehydration
- TVS suggestive of molar pregnancy

Management of hyperemesis

Rehydration, at least three litres of crystalloids initially.

Avoid glucose as it can precipitate Wernicke's encephalopathy.

Antiemetics: first line, Cyclizine; second line, Prochlorperazine; third line, Metoclopromide; fourth line, Domperidone/Ondansetron.

Vitamin supplementation especially Thiamine.

Role of corticosteroids in intractable hyperemesis.

Management of Molar pregnancy

Recommend suction curettage for confirmation of diagnosis by histology.

Discuss the preparations and planning before undertaking the surgical evacuation of uterus.

Discuss about referral to the regional trophoblastic screening centre for further management of molar pregnancy and follow up.

Discuss contraception: barrier methods until HCG levels revert to normal.

Further reading

The Management of Gestational Trophoblastic Disease, RCOG Green–top Guideline No. 38; February 2010. https://www.rcog.org.uk/globalassets/documents/guidelines/gt38managementgestational0210.pdf

The Management of Nausea and Vomiting of Pregnancy and Hyperemesis Gravidarum, RCOG Green-top Guideline No. 69 June 2016. https://www.rcog.org.uk/globalassets/documents/guidelines/green-top-guidelines/gtg69-hyperemesis.pdf

Task 4 **Miscarriage**

Instructions for Candidate

This task assesses the following clinical skills:

- Patient safety
- Communication with patients and their relatives
- Information gathering
- Applied clinical knowledge

Miss Elizabeth Barnes, 38 years, P_0, attended for her routine dating scan at 12^{+6} weeks. It was a natural conception and she's fit and healthy. After transabdominal scan, the sonographer checked with her if she was sure about her dates and referred her to the early pregnancy unit for a transvaginal scan. Elizabeth is sure about her last period and is understandably anxious and wants to know what's going on?

You are the registrar in early pregnancy clinic who scans Elizabeth. The scan is there for you to see and interpret. Your task is to:

- Interpret the scan findings
- Make a diagnosis
- Discuss management options with the patient

You have 10 minutes for this task (+ 2mins initial reading time).

Instructions for Assessor

This clinical assessment task is to assess the skills of the candidate to take a focussed history, interpret the scan findings, make a diagnosis and discuss the management options with the patient emphasising on shared decision making.

Give the candidates a few minutes (2) for focussed history taking.

Then present to them the scan pictures (Figures 17.2 and 17.3) and ask them what do they think is the diagnosis?

The next part of the station would be the interaction of the candidate with the role player focussing on discussion of management options and involving her in decision making.

Finally, record your overall clinical impression of the candidate (i.e. should this performance be a clear pass, borderline, or fail).

Instructions for Role Player

You are Elizabeth Barnes, 38 years of age. You have come to antenatal clinic for dating scan at 12^{+6} weeks into your first pregnancy. The scan doesn't show an ongoing healthy (viable) pregnancy corresponding to your dates and you are advised to have an internal scan (TVS), to date this pregnancy and make a diagnosis. You are very anxious as you are sure about your dates and know that something is not right.

It was a spontaneous conception; pregnancy test was positive 3 days after you missed your period. You've been taking Folic acid. You felt nauseous only during the first few weeks of pregnancy but recently you haven't experienced any nausea/vomiting or breast tenderness. You haven't had any bleeding and you thought that it was quite normal for the pregnancy symptoms to disappear after the first few weeks. You smoke 10–15/day but have been trying to cut down. You haven't had alcohol

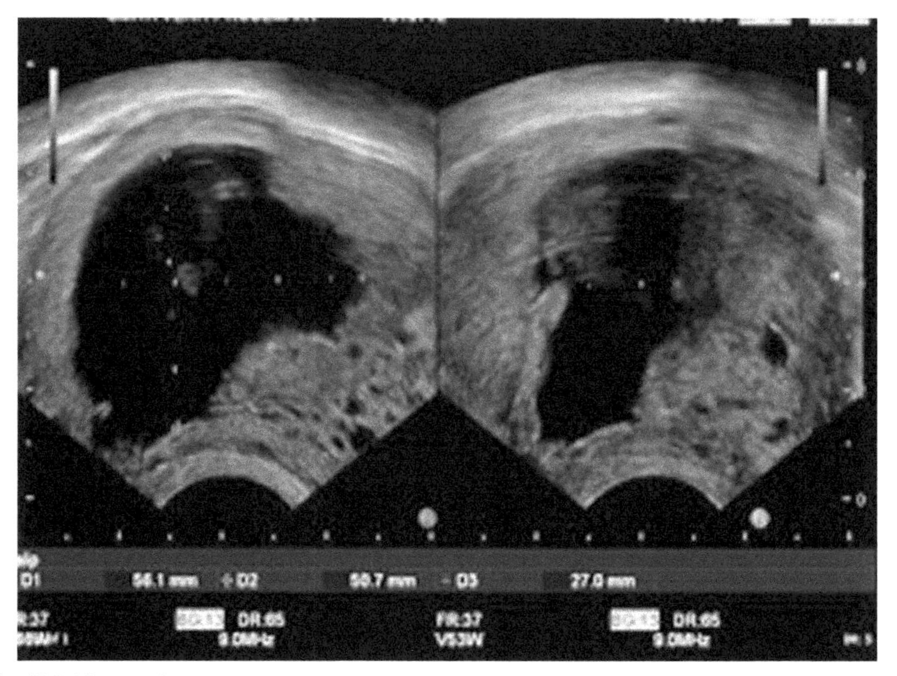

Fig. 17.2 Ultrasound

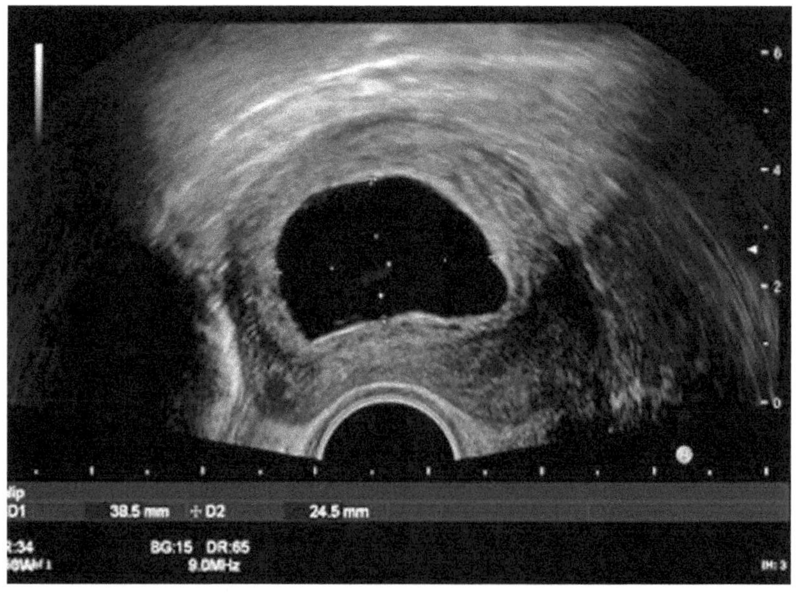

Fig. 17.3 Ultrasound

since being pregnant. You exercise regularly and you wonder if smoking or running five miles, three to four times per week may have caused your miscarriage. This was a planned pregnancy. You and your partner had been trying for nine months to get pregnant and you were not expecting this diagnosis. Hence you are taken aback by shock.

You are very upset and confirm with the doctor if they are sure about their diagnosis. After they confirm the diagnosis, you want to know your options. The doctor will discuss about expectant, medical and surgical options. You don't want to leave 'it' in you any longer and discard the expectant management. You are unsure about the other two options and want to know a bit more. You tell the candidate that a friend of yours had a major haemorrhage after having some tablets for miscarriage and she ended up in a hysterectomy. Could this happen to you? You want to know the risks of each option. You ask the doctor if they were in your place what would they do? You ask if the surgical option could affect your fertility. You also want to know if this could happen again to you and if miscarriage a common occurrence.

You ask the doctor how long you should wait before trying again. Is there anything that you would have done to avoid this miscarriage and is there anything that they would advise you to do differently next time? Should you have any investigations to know why it happened?

You feel calmer by the doctor's empathetic approach and if you get reasonable answers to your questions. You then say that you are still unsure and want to discuss with your partner. You expect the candidate to offer you written information and another appointment or contact numbers.

Assessment

Marking Scheme

Patient safety:

Pass	Borderline	Fail

Communication with patients and their relatives:

Pass	Borderline	Fail

Information gathering:

Pass	Borderline	Fail

Applied clinical knowledge:

Pass	Borderline	Fail

Notes for Marking

Patient safety

- Assesses patient's main concerns and ideas
- Gives options and discusses the pros and cons of each
- Involves patient in the process (e.g. encouraging them to express their ideas, or preferences)
- Negotiates a mutually agreed, acceptable and safe management plan
- Open and honest
- Offers an apology for delay in diagnosis and causing anxiety to the patient
- Gives honest and factual answers to the patient's queries

Communication with patients and their relatives

- Greets, introduces self and role, checks patient's name
- Consent to proceed **and** explains nature of interview
- Assesses patient's starting point (what the patient wants to know) **and** sets the agenda
- Empathetic approach
- Clear organized explanation in logical sequence
- Avoids use of medical jargon
- Avoids giving too much information at a time
- Checks patient's understanding
- Uses visual aids appropriately e.g. diagrams or uses analogies to aid explanation

Information gathering

- Obtains a focussed and relevant history
- Obtains patient's views, expectations, and concerns

Applied clinical knowledge

- Takes a focussed history
- Demonstrates a sound and comprehensive evidence-based clinical knowledge
- Counsels the patient with relevant information that is factually correct.
- Makes a safe management plan after offering all options

Notes for the Candidate

Focussed history taking

Take a brief and focussed history to explore the patient's background and establish rapport.

Interpret scan findings

Empty gestational sac with mean sac diameter > 25mm, suggestive of missed miscarriage.

Explanation of diagnosis to the patient

- 'It seems pregnancy stopped growing at a very early stage'
- Allow time for diagnosis to sink in
- 'Sometimes the usual symptoms of miscarriage like bleeding and pain do not present and hence it's called a missed miscarriage'
- Pause
- Allow patient to react and to lead
- Emphasize miscarriage is a common occurrence (incidence 20%)
- Ask if she wants anyone around her at this time
- Ask if it's appropriate to discuss management options at this stage

Discussion of management

- Discuss expectant, medical and surgical managements of miscarriage
- Discuss risks and benefits of each option
- Involve patient in decision making
- Don't impose what you may think is the right option for her
- Avoid using medical jargon

- Medical management successful in 9/10 cases but if it fails or there's a lot of bleeding, might need surgical option and hysterectomy is a rare but known complication
- Ensure surgical option unlikely to affect fertility unless there are any complications
- Ensure patient doesn't consider herself guilty for the event
- Could use phrases like 'nothing that you have done or could have done differently would have prevented it'
- Reassure >90% chances of a successful pregnancy outcome after a miscarriage
- No investigations indicated after a single miscarriage
- Allow at least one normal menstrual cycle before trying again but could start trying when feels physically and emotionally well
- Should take Folic acid at least a month before conception when planning next time

Closure

- Offer follow-up appointment to discuss further
- Offer written information and contact numbers
- Mention Miscarriage Association

Further reading

Ectopic pregnancy and miscarriage: diagnosis and initial management Clinical guideline [CG154] Published date: December 2012. https://www.nice.org.uk/guidance/cg154?unlid=10289279720161020201 21

Chapter 18 **Gynaecological Oncology**

Task 1 **Cervical cytology**

Instructions for Candidate

This task assesses the following clinical skills:

- Patient safety
- Communication with patients and their relatives
- Information gathering
- Applied clinical knowledge

Your consultant has asked you to speak to Agnieska Polanski aged 38 whose smear result has shown 'severe dyskaryosis', HPV positive.

Your task is to:

- break the news to Agnieska about the abnormal smear
- discuss the next stage of management (i.e. colposcopy and biopsy)
- answer any questions

You do not need to take a history.

You have 10 minutes for this task (+ 2mins initial reading time).

Instructions for Assessor

Please read the instructions for candidates and actors.

This station is designed to test the candidate's ability to break bad news in a sensitive and professional way. This case involves a patient who has a severely abnormal cervical smear result (with the possibility of early cervical cancer). The candidate explains the implications of such a smear and discusses the next step in management.

Record your overall clinical impression of the candidate for each domain (e.g. should this performance be pass, borderline, or a fail.

Instructions for Role Player

You are Agnieska Polanski, aged 38 years, and you have come to an outpatient gynaecology clinic (called a colposcopy clinic) to discuss your recent cervical smear result. You have a feeling that the smear might be abnormal because the secretary refused to discuss it with you on the phone and you received a very prompt appointment to see the doctor.

You love children and work part time in a local nursery and after school club whilst you are studying for a NVQ level 3 childcare qualification. Your social life is great at the moment—you live with a very supportive and loving partner Lee and are planning to get married next year. Your partner and you have planned to have children and you will probably come off the pill just before your wedding (because at your age you don't want to leave it too long but you don't want to look huge in your wedding dress).

You haven't had regular smears for a while, but decided you would get a check up because you wanted to be 'checked over' before starting a family. You were very surprised that you have been called back and have no symptoms or clues that there might have been anything wrong. When you are told there is a problem with the smear you will be very shocked. You hadn't really realized that 'abnormal smear' could be leading to cancer. Everyone seemed so relaxed about it before and now they are talking about an operation! You do not know much about abnormal cells in cervical smears—you had a friend who was called back for another smear but it was all a false alarm and there was nothing wrong on her repeat smear. You kind of hope this might be a false alarm as well.

You are worried about developing cancer, but are also worried that if there is something wrong it might mean that you will have trouble getting pregnant or even worse—not be able to have children at all.

Once you get over the shock of the diagnosis you ask about the next step in your treatment. You are recommended to have a colposcopy (look at cervix) and a biopsy from your cervix and want to have this explained as well. However, the doctor may say they need to ask the consultant to see you to give you further details—you will accept this, providing they are sympathetic and clear.

Key concerns

- Is this cancer or not?
- What does 'Positive for HPV mean'? Can this infection be treated?
- What does the investigation involve?
- Could treatment affect your potential for having children in the future?

Assessment

Marking Scheme

Patient safety:

Pass Borderline Fail

Communication with patients and their relatives:

Pass Borderline Fail

Information gathering:

Pass Borderline Fail

Applied clinical knowledge:

Pass Borderline Fail

Notes for Marking

Patient safety

- Assesses the patient's main concerns
- Involves patient in the process (e.g. encouraging them to express their ideas, or preferences)
- Aware of the correlation between HPV and cervical dyskaryosis/CIN/Ca
- Negotiates a mutually agreed acceptable, safe, plan
- Open and honest about the abnormal smear result without being patronising

- Open and honest about the risk of invasive disease if untreated
- Avoids platitudes or false re-assurance

Communication with patients and their relatives

- Greets patient and obtains patient's name
- Introduces self, role
- Explains nature of interview (reason for coming to talk to patient)
- Assesses starting point: what patient understands already/is feeling
- Gives clear signposting that serious important information is to follow
- Chunks and checks, using patient's response to guide next steps
- Discovers what other information would help the patient, attempts to address patient's information needs
- Gives explanation in an organized manner (signposting/summarising)
- Uses clear language, avoids jargon and confusing language
- Picks up and responds to patient's non-verbal cues
- Allows patient time to react (use of silence, allows for shut-down)
- Recognizes, acknowledges and validates patient's concerns and feelings (e.g. uses empathy)
- Appropriate non-verbal behaviour e.g. eye contact, posture and position, movement, facial expression, use of voice (pace, tone)
- Provides support: e.g. concern, understanding, willingness to help

Information gathering

- Obtains relevant history regarding cervical smears
- Obtains patients expectations and concerns regarding starting a family as well as the possibility of cancer

Applied clinical knowledge

- Demonstrates a sound and comprehensive evidence-based clinical knowledge
- Explanation of problem—(abnormal cells, precancerous—might lead to invasive disease if not treated)
- HPV—these are in fact a large family of viruses, only a few of which are involved in causing abnormalities of the cervix and lower genital tract. Of the over 150 HPV viruses, the main types responsible for changes to the cervix are types 16, 18, 31, 33, and 45. About four out of five adult men and women have had HPV infection at some time in their lives, but only a small minority of women with an HPV infection ultimately have an abnormal smear and a tiny fraction of these get cervical cancer. It is acquired in almost all cases through close intimate or sexual contact,
- No antibiotics or other treatment for HPV infection is required.
- Fertility—no effect on fertility
- Explains colposcopy—(detailed examination of the neck of the womb done via speculum. A colposcope is a magnifying glass, which allows examination of cell changes on the cervix. Sometimes video equipment is used so patient can view the examination on a screen if she wishes)
- Explains about the procedure—a biopsy will be needed to see how abnormal the cells are, and how far they extend into the neck of womb
- Explains that this will be needed for deciding about further treatment
- May discuss see and treat with LLETZ (Large Loop Excision of Transformation Zone). Some candidates may mention about cone biopsy

Notes for Candidate

Please read Chapter 2 about the five communication skills principles of Calgary –Cambridge model of communication theory.

Further reading

Familiarise yourself with the BSCCP recommendations. https://www.bsccp.org.uk

Task 2 **Postmenopausal bleeding**

Instructions for Candidate

This task assesses the following clinical skills:

- Patient safety
- Communication with patients and their relatives
- Information gathering
- Applied clinical knowledge

You are the Registrar in the clinic.

Your next patient Mrs. Valerie Cameron is a 60-year-old woman with a BMI of 53. She is a diabetic and hypertensive. She has three children.

She had been seen in the postmenopausal bleeding clinic two weeks ago. Her pelvic ultrasound had shown the endometrial thickness to be 8mm. Endometrial sample was obtained which has shown hyperplasia without atypia.

Your task is to explain the endometrial biopsy and make a management plan (six minutes). You will then be provided some data to explain to Valerie and organise further management plan (six mins).

You have 10 minutes for this task (+ 2mins initial reading time).

Instructions for Assessor

This clinical assessment task assesses the candidate's ability to explain complex medical terminology in simple lay terms to the patient. It also addresses the candidate's ability to address the wider health issues—in this case obesity and diabetes.

As this lady is at high risk of endometrial cancer and will refuse an intrauterine system, she will need treatment with oral progesterone for six months and then a repeat biopsy at six months, to be repeated in six months and then annually.

This clinical assessment task consists of two consultations.

The first for explanation and planning of hyperplasia without atypia and the second for hyperplasia with atypia, Give six minutes each.

At the second biopsy, (one year from now), the histology shows hyperplasia with atypia. The candidates are expected to explain this to Valerie and explain the management plan. If the candidates have not made a plan for the second six monthly endometrial sampling, tell them that their consultant had reviewed the notes and organised the repeat biopsy and then tell them the result.

Record your overall clinical impression of the candidate for each domain (e.g. should this performance be pass, borderline, or a fail).

Instructions for Royal Player

You are Valerie Cameron, a 60-year-old woman. You run the local fish and chip shop with your partner.

You have had bleeding for just two days about three weeks ago.

You were not worried as the bleeding was not heavy and stopped on its own. You were having a conversation with one your regular customers that you thought your periods are over but then you get one. The customer told you to report this to your GP as this is how her sister's cancer of the womb was diagnosed.

You therefore made a GP appointment, the next day you had the scan and the day after you were in the hospital clinic.

The doctor who saw you in the clinic (was called postmenopausal bleeding clinic) took a biopsy from the lining of the womb. You found that very painful and brought tears to your eyes.

You have always been a big girl and are now tired of people telling you to reduce weight. You are very busy and do not have time to make fancy salads. Any way you do not think you eat too much. You are working all throughout the day, how much more exercise can a person do?

Anyway, your already have diabetes which is controlled with medications. Every one in your family has had raised blood pressure, so it is unlikely to be related to your weight.

You have come on your own as your husband has to look after the shop work.

Ideas: You have an idea that the appointment is to discuss the biopsy result as that is what your clinic appointment letter has said both the times

Concerns: You are now concerned that it could be cancer, just like the sister of your customer had. You are terrified and are now repenting come alone.

You also are concerned that they might do another biopsy and you really do not want that.

You are also completely opposed to the treatment with a coil (Intrauterine system). You will therefore choose the option of taking the progesterone tablets.

When told that you will require repeat biopsies, ask why could you just not have a hysterectomy?

When you are told that the biopsy a year later has shown progression, say 'I was telling you to do a hysterectomy a year earlier and then this would not have happened'.

Expectations: You expect the doctor to explain to you what exactly the biopsy means. What are the chances of cancer developing and what are the means to prevent that and how will it be tested?

At the second consultation, you want to know what further management plan would be.

Assessment

Marking Scheme

Patient safety:

Pass	Borderline	Fail

Communication with patients and their relatives:

Pass	Borderline	Fail

Information gathering:

Pass	Borderline	Fail

Applied clinical knowledge:

Pass	Borderline	Fail

Notes for Marking

Patient safety

- Assesses the patient's main concerns and ideas
- Gives options and discusses the pros and cons of each
- Involves patient in the process (e.g. encouraging them to express their ideas, or preferences)
- Negotiates a mutually agreed acceptable, safe, plan
- Open and honest about complications

- Honest discussion about the importance of weight loss and health life style
- Avoids platitudes or false re-assurance

Communication with patients and their relatives

- Greets patient and obtains patient's name
- Introduces self, role
- Explains nature of interview (reason for coming to talk to patient)
- Assesses starting point: what patient understands already/is feeling
- Gives clear signposting that serious important information is to follow
- Chunks and checks, using patient's response to guide next steps
- Discovers what other information would help the patient, attempts to address patient's information needs
- Gives explanation in an organised manner (signposting/summarising)
- Uses clear language, avoids jargon and confusing language
- Picks up and responds to patient's non-verbal cues
- Allows patient time to react (use of silence, allows for shut-down)
- Recognises, acknowledges and validates patient's concerns and feelings (e.g. uses empathy)
- Appropriate non-verbal behaviour e.g. eye contact, posture and position, movement, facial expression, use of voice (pace, tone)
- Provides support: e.g. concern, understanding, willingness to help
- Language (easily understood, avoids or explains jargon)
- Uses visual aids appropriately e.g. diagrams, or uses analogies to aid explanation
- Avoids platitudes or false reassurance

Information gathering

- Obtains relevant history regarding postmenopausal bleeding and any risk factors for ca endometrium
- Obtains patients expectations and concerns

Applied clinical knowledge Tasks 1 and 2

- Demonstrates a sound and comprehensive evidence-based clinical knowledge
- Counsels the patient with relevant information that is factually correct.
- Makes a robust and safe management plan
- Aware of management of hyperplasia with and without atypia
- Educates patient about life style changes to mitigate risk factors

Notes for Candidates

Please familiarise yourself with the different situations for patients presenting with endometrial hyperplasia, i.e. Pre- and post-menopausal patients. Patients that are wishing for fertility etc.

Explanation of hyperplasia without atypia:

- In a simple way without using medical jargon e.g. thickening of the lining of the womb due to rapid growth of the lining cells, without any abnormality in the structure of the cell
- Use pen and paper to draw schematically to explain

Risk of progression to endometrial cancer:

- The risk of endometrial hyperplasia without atypia progressing to endometrial cancer is less than 5% over 20 years and that the majority of cases of endometrial hyperplasia without atypia will regress spontaneously during follow-up

Management of hyperplasia without atypia:

- Both continuous oral and local intrauterine (levonorgestrel-releasing intrauterine system [LNG-IUS]) progestogens are effective in achieving regression of endometrial hyperplasia without atypia
- The LNG-IUS should be the first-line medical treatment because compared with oral progestogens it has a higher disease regression rate with a more favourable bleeding profile and it is associated with fewer adverse effects
- Continuous progestogens should be used (medroxyprogesterone 10–20 mg/day or norethisterone 10–15mg/day) for women who decline the LNG-IUS
- Cyclical progestogens should not be used because they are less effective in inducing regression of endometrial hyperplasia without atypia compared with continuous oral progestogens or the LNG-IUS
- Treatment with oral progestogens or the LNG-IUS should be for a minimum of 6 months in order to induce histological regression of endometrial hyperplasia without atypia.
- Hysterectomy should not be conidered as a first-line treatment for hyperplasia without atypia because progestogen therapy induces histological and symptomatic remission in the majority of women and avoids the morbidity associated with major surgery especially with a high BMI and co-morbidities

Explains the high risk factors in this patient:

- Further surveillance: endometrial surveillance incorporating outpatient endometrial biopsy is recommended after a diagnosis of hyperplasia without atypia
- Endometrial surveillance should be arranged at a minimum of six-monthly intervals, although review schedules should be individualised and responsive to changes in a woman's clinical condition
- At least two consecutive six-monthly negative biopsies should be obtained prior to discharge. Women should be advised to seek a further referral if abnormal vaginal bleeding recurs after completion of treatment because this may indicate disease relapse
- In women at higher risk of relapse, such as women with a body mass index (BMI) of 35 or greater or those treated with oral progestogens, six-monthly endometrial biopsies are recommended. Once two consecutive negative endometrial biopsies have been obtained then long-term follow-up should be considered with annual endometrial biopsy

Referral to obesity services/dietician:

- Endometrial hyperplasia is often associated with multiple identifiable risk factors and assessment should aim to identify and monitor these factors
- This patient may qualify for Bariatric surgery

Task 2

Explanation of hyperplasia with atypia:

- In a simple way without using medical jargon e.g. thickening of the lining of the womb due to rapid growth of the lining cells, with abnormality in the structure of the cell
- Use pen and paper to draw schematically to explain

Risk of progression to endometrial cancer and associated endometrial cancer:

The risk of developing endometrial cancer is highest in hyperplasia with atypia. Women diagnosed with hyperplasia with atypia found that the cumulative risk of cancer in four years was 8% which increased to 12.4% after nine years and to 27.5% after 19 years.

Hyperplasia with atypia has also been associated with a rate of concomitant carcinoma of up to 43% in women undergoing hysterectomy.

Management of hyperplasia with atypia:

- Women with hyperplasia with atypia should undergo a total hysterectomy because of the risk of underlying malignancy or progression to cancer
- A laparoscopic approach to total hysterectomy is preferable to an abdominal approach as it is associated with a shorter hospital stay, less postoperative pain and quicker recovery
- In this patient a laparoscopic assisted vaginal hysterectomy with bilateral salpingo-oophorectomy could be offered
- There is no benefit from intraoperative frozen section analysis of the endometrium or routine lymphadenectomy
- Postmenopausal women with hyperplasia with atypia should be offered bilateral salpingo-oophorectomy together with the total hysterectomy

Further reading

Green-top Guideline No. 67 RCOG/BSGE Joint Guideline | February 2016. https://www.rcog.org.uk/globalassets/documents/guidelines/green-top-guidelines/gtg_67_endometrial_hyperplasia.pdf

Task 3 **Ovarian cancer**

Instructions for Candidate

This task assesses the following clinical skills:

- Patient safety
- Communication with patients and their relatives
- Information gathering
- Applied clinical knowledge

You are a ST5 doctor in the gynaecology clinic. You are asked to see Jane Reynolds who is a 60-year-old lady. She has been referred by her GP. She presented with non-specific mild symptoms of abdominal bloating and reduced appetite. The GP organised some investigations including a blood test and a scan. The CA-125 has been reported as 18 iu/L. An ultrasound scan shows a unilateral ovarian cyst measuring 10cm. The cyst has some small solid areas and multi-cystic areas. There is no ascites.

You will have ten minutes for the history taking and explanation of investigations. The patient has already been told by the GP that this may be a cancer, so it is not a breaking-bad-news station. Once you have finished the discussion with Jane the assessor will ask you some questions.

You have 10 minutes for this task (+ 2mins initial reading time).

Instructions for Assessor

Please read the instruction for the candidate and actor.

After the consultation between the candidate and patient actor comes to an end (or in the last four minutes), tell the candidate that Jane underwent a laparoscopic bilateral salpingo-oophorectomy, and the histology confirmed ovarian cancer within one ovary.

Ask the candidate to explain to Jane about the next surgical and medical treatments suitable for her diagnosis.

There are some marks on the process mark sheet for the actor to assign at the end of the station.

Record your overall clinical impression of the candidate for each domain (i.e. should this performance be pass, borderline, or a fail).

Instructions for Role Player

You are Jane Reynolds, a 60-year-old retired nurse. You had previously been very well, but noticed some mild intermittent abdominal bloating, a reduced appetite, and occasional diarrhoea over the last six months. You had put it down to irritable bowel syndrome (IBS) or diverticular disease, from which you've suffered in the past. You are otherwise normally well, and have never had any operations. You do not take any medication. You don't smoke or drink. Your grandmother died of ovarian cancer in her 60s and your sister and niece have both had breast cancer under the age of 40.

You have been sent for a blood test called CA-125 but you do not yet know the result. The radiographer told you that there was a cyst on your ovary. Your GP has already told you over the phone that there is a possibility that this may be a cancer, hence she's referring you to hospital.

Temperament: You are generally a calm, level-headed woman and used to be a nurse, so know a bit about ovaries and gynaecological problems already.

Ideas: Initially you thought that this was just down to your IBS or diverticular disease, but since you've looked on the internet, you have read about the risk of ovarian cancer in post-menopausal women. You also briefly read about the risk of breast and ovarian cancer running in families.

Concerns: You want to know what needs to be done about this cyst and how quickly it can be treated. You presume you need an operation. If this is a cancer, you want to know whether there is a risk your daughters may have inherited anything, and whether they are at risk also.

Expectations: Having had the conversation with your GP about the fact this could possibly be ovarian cancer, you want to have a plan for your management. You already know that this is possibly bad news.

You want the doctor to explain:

- What does the blood test mean?
- Are there any other suitable blood tests? You've read about other blood tests for ovarian cancer.
- What concerning features are looked for on an ultrasound scan of the ovaries and pelvis? Do you have any of these concerning features?
- How can the doctors predict whether this is a cancer or not?
- What other investigations may be necessary?
- What operation is recommended?
- Is there a timescale, according to national guidelines, by which this operation should be done?
- If this is a cancer, will you need any other operations or treatment afterwards?

You had a laparoscopic bilateral salpingo-oophorectomy, and the histology confirms ovarian cancer within one ovary. After the assessor has provided the candidate with this information, you have some further questions to ask. These include:

- What further surgery would be recommended to complete my treatment?
- What other non-surgical treatment might I need?
- What sort of investigations or referrals may be available to test whether my family is at risk of cancer?

At the end there are some marks for you to award according to how well the candidate explained your questions and concerns.

Assessment

Marking Scheme

Patient safety:

Pass Borderline Fail

Communication with patients and their relatives:

Pass Borderline Fail

Information gathering:

Pass Borderline Fail

Applied clinical knowledge:

Pass Borderline Fail

Notes for Marking

Patient safety

- Assesses patient's main concerns and ideas
- Gives recommendation for surgery

- Involves patient in the process (e.g. encouraging them to express their ideas, or preferences)
- Negotiates a mutually agreed, acceptable, and safe management plan

Communication with patients and their relatives

- Greets, introduces self and role, checks patient's name
- Consent to proceed and explains nature of interview
- Structured, concise history-taking of valid points
- Assesses patient's starting point (what the patient already knows and wants to know) and sets the agenda
- Clear organised explanation in logical sequence
- Chunks: i.e. provides information in reasonable chunks
- Check patient's understanding.
- Language (easily understood, avoids or explains jargon)
- Uses visual aids appropriately e.g. diagrams or uses analogies to aid explanation

Information gathering

- Obtains relevant history regarding her presenting symptoms
- Obtains patients expectations and concerns regarding the diagnosis or treatment of cancer of the ovary

Applied clinical knowledge

- Demonstrates a sound and comprehensive evidence-based clinical knowledge.
- Counsels the patient with relevant information that is factually correct.
- Makes a robust and safe management plan.
- Recommends and calculates the RMI to calculate risk.

Notes for Candidate

History taking

- Common symptoms of ovarian cancer: bloating, change in bowel habit, weight loss, early satiety, abdominal pain, urinary symptoms. New symptoms of IBS over the age of 50
- Past medical history: diverticular disease and IBS. This may have delayed her presentation of symptoms even longer
- Social history—relevance of nursing background, aids in identifying background knowledge before information-giving
- Family history—strong family history suggests BRCA inheritance and suitability for genetic referral
- Ideas, concerns and expectations; already knows of a probable diagnosis of cancer, thanks to the GP. It is important to know your patient's starting point before information-giving (i.e. no need for breaking bad news in this station)

Explanation of investigations

- CA-125 is a tumour maker blood test, often raised in epithelial ovarian cancers. However, it has been reported to only be raised in 50% of early stage ovarian malignancies
- In women under 40 with suspected ovarian cancer other blood tests should be performed. These include alpha fetoprotein (AFP), beta-human chorionic gonadotrophin (beta-hCG) and lactate dehydrogenase (LDH). However, in this case, because of the patient's age, these tests are not recommended or necessary

- Features of or predictive scores for ovarian cysts:
  - Features or characteristics of cysts seen on ultrasound scanning are often categorised as normal or suspicious. There are various models to predict the risk of malignancy. These include the Risk of Malignancy index (RMI) and the International Ovarian Tumour Analysis Group (IOTA). Both of these are recommended in the RCOG Greentop Guidelines.
- The **Risk of Malignancy Index** (RMI): **U x M x Ca-125**
  - **U** = USS features: The abnormal features noted on the RMI score include bilateral cysts, ascites, multi-locular cysts, solid features and the presence of metastases
    - The ultrasound result is scored 1 point for each of the characteristics. U = 0(USS of 0), U = 1 (for USS of 1); U = 3 (for USS score of 2-5)
  - **M** = Menopausal status. This is scored as 1 = premenopausal and 3 = post-menopausal
  - Serum CA-125 is measured in IU/ml
  - **Low** risk RMI score (< 25). This suggests < 3% risk of cancer. Management can be performed in a general gynaecology unit. Simple cysts < 5 cm with a Ca-125 may be managed conservatively, with 4-6/12-ly USS and Ca-125 for a year. Laparoscopic salpingo-oophorectomy is also acceptable
  - **Moderate** risk RMI score (25-250). This suggests a 20% risk of cancer. These women should be managed in a cancer unit. Laparoscopic oophorectomy is recommended, and full surgical staging if a cancer is diagnosed
  - **High** risk RMI score (>250). This suggests > 75% risk of cancer. Management should be in a cancer centre. Full staging should be performed. Some units perform frozen section on the pelvic mass, and await results before proceeding straight to full surgical staging
- **IOTA** score
  - This divides ultrasound features into benign and malignant. Any malignant features require referral to a gynaecological oncology service
  - **Benign** features: unilocular cysts, solid components where the largest solid component is < 7 mm, acoustic shadowing, smooth multilocular tumour with a diameter < 100mm, no blood flow
  - **Malignant** features: irregular solid tumour, ascites, at least four papillary structures, irregular multilocular solid tumour with diameter ≥100mm, very strong blood flow

Initial treatment plan

- Mrs Reynolds results should be discussed at the cancer unit's multidisciplinary team (MDT) meeting
- Mrs Reynolds has a moderate RMI score. RMI = 162
- She should be offered a laparoscopic bilateral salpingo-oophorectomy
- It is recommended that she should have both ovaries removed. This is because she is already post-menopausal, and because of the risk of disease in the other ovary
- Every effort should be made to avoid rupture of the cyst during laparoscopic removal. The use of a laparoscopic bag e.g. eco-sac, is recommended to avoid intra-abdominal cyst contents spillage. If spillage does occur, and the cyst is found to be malignant, the FIGO stage is affected
- If laparoscopic removal is considered too difficult or risk of rupture is too high, mini-laparotomy can be performed

- According to NICE guidelines:
  - All women being referred with suspected ovarian malignancy should be seen within two weeks of referral
  - All women should receive their treatment within 31 days from the decision to treat date
- If a patient is found to have a HIGH RMI score, (i.e. > 75% risk of cancer)
  - The patient should be investigated further with a CT of the abdomen and pelvis. This is for radiological staging. If there are clinical concerns or if the initial CT suggests malignant disease, she should also have a chest CT to look for further pulmonary metastatic disease. MRI is not appropriate in this situation. MRI is normally used for characterising ovarian cysts
  - The patient should be treated with a full laparotomy and staging procedure. This will be discussed below

Treatment plan after histological results

- Mrs Reynold's results should be discussed at the MDT meeting again
- To gain further information, Mrs Reynolds should be offered a full laparotomy and staging procedure. A gynaecological oncology surgeon, in a cancer centre, should perform this. This involves:
  - Extended midline laparotomy
  - Cytology (ascites or washings)
  - Biopsies from adhesions and suspicious areas
  - Total abdominal hysterectomy
  - Omental biopsy
  - Bilateral salpingo-oophorectomy (if not already completed)
  - Retroperitoneal lymph node assessment (pelvic and para-aortic)
- NICE recommends pelvic and para-aortic lymph node 'assessment'. They do not recommend systematic retroperitoneal lymphadenectomy (block dissection of lymph nodes from the pelvic side walls to the level of the renal vein) as part of standard surgical treatment. There are differing opinions within the gynaecological oncology specialty. Some units do perform full lymphadenectomy as part of their staging procedures
- Adjuvant systemic chemotherapy
  - If Mrs Reynolds is 'fully staged' and found to only have low risk stage 1 disease (grade 1 or 2, stage 1a or 1b), it is not recommended that she receive chemotherapy
  - If Mrs Reynolds is 'fully staged' and found to have high-risk stage 1 disease (grade 3 or stage 1c), adjuvant chemotherapy is recommended. This consists of six cycles of carboplatin.
  - If Mrs Reynolds is 'fully staged' and found to have advanced ovarian cancer (stage II to IV), it is recommended that she receive double agent chemotherapy

Geneticist referrals

- Many cancer units routinely refer their patients with ovarian cancer to geneticists for assessment. This is often part of clinical trial criteria. In view of her family and personal history of ovarian and breast cancer, Mrs Reynolds is eligible for referral to specialist genetic counselling services. If after further family history, histological follow up from the cancer registry etc, the geneticists will decide on her suitability for BRCA testing
- NICE 2013 guidelines 'Familial breast cancer: classification, care and managing breast cancer and related risks in people with a family history of breast cancer' (CG164) have many criteria regarding referral to secondary care or geneticist assessment
- Regarding her daughters, they meet the following criteria and should be offered a referral to a specialist genetic clinic:

- Families containing one relative with ovarian cancer at any age and, on the same side of the family:
  - One first-degree relative (including the relative with ovarian cancer) or second-degree relative diagnosed with breast cancer at younger age than 50 years, **or**
  - Two first-degree or second-degree relatives diagnosed with breast cancer at younger than an average age of 60 years **or**
  - Another ovarian cancer at any age

Further reading

Ovarian cancer: recognition and initial management. NICE guideline (CG122). Published April 2011. https://www.nice.org.uk/guidance/cg122

Ovarian cysts in postmenopausal women. Royal College of Obstetricians and Gynaecologists' Green-top Guideline number 34. Published October 2003, reviewed 2010. https://www.rcog.org.uk/globalassets/documents/guidelines/gtg_62.pdf

Management of suspected ovarian masses in premenopausal women. Royal College of Obstetricians and Gynaecologists/British Society of Gynaecological Endoscopy Guideline Number 62. Published July 2016. https://www.rcog.org.uk/globalassets/documents/guidelines/green-top-guidelines/gtg_34.pdf

Task 4 **Vulval intraepithelial neoplasia (VIN)**

Instructions for Candidate

This task assesses the following clinical skills:

- Patient safety
- Communication with patients and their relatives
- Information gathering
- Applied clinical knowledge

Amanda Rogers is a 35-year-old lady who was seen in the gynaecology clinic two weeks ago. She had presented with a history of vulval itching and burning around the vulva. On examination she had an irregular pigmented plaque on the right labia. This was biopsied.

Amanda is on immunosuppressive medication following her renal transplant two years back. She had three children all born vaginally before her transplant. She had a Mirena IUS *in-situ* and has no periods. She is on yearly smears in view of her history. She also had a LLETZ procedure for CIN3 last year. Last smear was normal.

The biopsy has detected high grade vulval squamous intraepithelial lesion (SIL) also called vulval intraepithelial neoplasia (VIN).

You are the registrar in the Gynaecology clinic and Amanda has her follow up appointment today to discuss the results and further treatment options

You have 10 minutes for this task (+ 2mins initial reading time).

Instructions for Assessor

Please read instructions to candidate and actor.

Record your overall clinical impression of the candidate for each domain (e.g. should this performance be pass, borderline, or a fail).

Instructions for Role Player

You are Amanda Rogers a 35-year-old accountant. You are here to receive the vulval biopsy result which was taken on the last visit.

You had three children in the past all were normal births. You have a Mirena coil for the last four years. Your periods have stopped all together.

You are a non-smoker. You had a renal transplant two years back and since then you are feeling great.

The vulval itching has been brothering you for a year. Sometimes you have burning sensation in the vulval area. You are also worried that itching is not settling and the area can be sore for a while. Furthermore as you had the biopsy last time and you are quite convinced that it may be a bad news.

Temperament: You just want to get on with your life as you feel well after the transplant.

Ideas: You are hoping that the treatment by the doctor will cure it all together

Concerns: You want to know whether its cancer. Is there a treatment to get rid of the condition? You want your life back. The changes in the smear test followed by LLETZ treatment last year have made you worried that condition may be spreading to the skin on the outside. You are worried that you may give it to you husband.

Expectations: You want the doctor to explain what it is and what's the cause?
What the treatment involves and how long should she use it for?
Will it spread to the rest of your body?
What are the other complications? Can it turn into cancer?

Assessment

Marking Scheme		
Patient safety:		
Pass	Borderline	Fail
Communication with patients and their relatives:		
Pass	Borderline	Fail
Information gathering:		
Pass	Borderline	Fail
Applied clinical knowledge:		
Pass	Borderline	Fail

Notes for Marking

Patient safety

- Assesses the patient's main concerns and ideas
- Discusses possible treatment options and associated complications
- Involves patient in the process (e.g. encouraging them to express their ideas, or preferences)
- Negotiates a mutually agreed acceptable, safe, plan
- Open and honest about the diagnosis of pre cancer and the risk of malignant transformation if left untreated
- Provides with information about VIN and SIL e.g. information leaflet; support from specialist nurses

Communication with patients and their relatives

- Greets, introduces self and role, checks patient's name
- Consent to proceed and explains nature of interview
- Assesses patient's starting point (what the patient wants to know) and sets the agenda
- Clear organised explanation in logical sequence
- Chunks: e.g. provides information in reasonable chunks
- Checks patient's understanding.
- Language (easily understood, avoids or explains jargon)

Information gathering

- Obtains relevant history regarding her presenting symptoms of vulval itching
- Obtains patients expectations and concerns

Applied clinical knowledge

- Demonstrates a sound and comprehensive evidence-based clinical knowledge as previously documented

Notes for Candidate

The scenario is taken from a common clinical scenario of our daily practice. It not only assesses the process of communication but also assesses the content of the knowledge given to the patient. It is important *how* you provide the information to the patient.

In counselling Ms Rogers, the candidates must include the following:

- VIN/SIL is a precancerous skin lesion of any part of the vulva. It is divided into two types—usual, which is HPV related (subdivided to wart, basaloid, and mixed), and differentiated, which has non-viral aetiology
- It is not cancer but vulval squamous cell cancer occurs in about 15% of women if VIN/SIL is left untreated
- VIN/SIL may occur in women of all ages. The following factors have been associated with VIN/SIL
  - HPV causes half of all cases of VIN/SIL. It also causes other genital precancerous lesions or cancers involving cervix, vagina, and anus
  - Smoking
  - Immunosuppression
  - Vulval inflammatory skin conditions particularly lichen sclerosus or erosive lichen planus
- Treatment options include:
  - Wide local excision
  - Skinning vulvectomy
  - Laser ablation
  - Topical treatment (e.g. Imiquimod)
- Careful follow-up after treatment is essential long term. VIN/SIL may recur, particularly if excision margins are inadequate. Follow-up every six to 12 months is recommended for at least five years after surgery for VIN/SIL.
- Up to 50% of women with VIN/SIL develop cervical intraepithelial neoplasia (CIN), anal intraepithelial neoplasia (AIN), vaginal intraepeithelial neoplasia (VAIN) or invasive cancer of the genital tract or anus. It is particularly important to have regular cervical smears

Practice this scenario with one of your friends who can act as a role player and ask another friend to provide you with feedback. We recommend you read the following:

Further reading

Powell JJ, Wojnarowska F. Lichen sclerosus. *Lancet*, 1999. 353: 1777–83.

Royal College of Obstetricians and Gynaecologist. The Management of Vulval Skin Disorders. Green-Top Guideline No. 58. London: RCOG; 2011.

Task 5 **Endometrial cancer**

Instructions for Candidate

This task assesses the following clinical skills:

- Patient safety
- Communication with patients and their relatives
- Information gathering
- Applied clinical knowledge

Your consultant has asked you to speak to Violet Morris, 74, who presented with postmenopausal bleeding. Endometrial biopsy shows low-grade adenocarcinoma.

Your task is to:

- Break the news to Violet about the abnormal result
- Respond appropriately to her reaction and address any concerns that she might have
- Give information about next stage of management

You do not need to take a history or agree a management plan.

You have 10 minutes for this task (+ 2mins initial reading time).

Instructions for Assessor

This station is designed to test the student's ability to break bad news in a sensitive and professional way. This case involves a patient who had presented with postmenopausal bleeding and the endometrial biopsy has shown endometrial cancer.

Do not interrupt the candidate unless they are not completing the task in which you may show them the candidate instructions again.

Record your overall clinical impression of the candidate for each domain (e.g. should this performance be pass, borderline, or a fail).

Instruction for Role Player

You are Violet Morris 74, and you have come to an outpatient gynaecology clinic to find out the result of the recent biopsy from your womb lining. You were seen in the clinic ten days ago for vaginal bleeding after the menopause. In clinic you had an ultrasound examination and a biopsy was taken from the lining of your womb. You have a feeling that the result might be abnormal because the secretary refused to discuss it with you on the phone and you received a very prompt appointment to see the doctor. Although they were very kind and helpful you could tell they were being evasive about the actual results.

You have been very busy recently looking after your husband George who had heart surgery (coronary artery bypass graft, CABG). He is still quite frail and dependent on you to look after him and as a result you had neglected to report the vaginal bleeding for some time.

You are worried that the biopsy might have shown cancer, and feel guilty for having neglected the symptoms. Even though you feel prepared for the worst you will be quiet and shocked when the candidate gives you the bad news. You will be sad, not angry. After a minute or two you get over the shock of the diagnosis you ask about what will happen next. Your main concerns are that you need to be at home with your husband. Who will look after George if you have to go in for an operation? You have no children and although you have lived in the same house for many years and have many friends in the community, you know George will not want them to come and look after him.

You are recommended to have some more investigations including a MRI scan but you don't know what this actually involves. The candidate explains that you will need surgery to remove your womb and ovaries. Again this will be quite bad news and will take a while to sink in—one of your neighbours had a hysterectomy last year and took months to recover.

The candidate may say they need to ask the consultant to see you to give you further details—you will accept this, providing they are sympathetic and clear.

Key concerns:

- What do the investigations involve? Why are they required?
- What does the surgery involve?
- Who will look after your husband if you are in hospital? You are very worried that he might have another heart attack with the news of the cancer

Assessment

Marking Scheme

Patient safety:

Pass Borderline Fail

Communication with patients and their relatives:

Pass Borderline Fail

Information gathering:

Pass Borderline Fail

Applied clinical knowledge:

Pass Borderline Fail

Notes for Marking

Patient safety

- Assesses the patient's main concerns
- Involves patient in the process (e.g. encouraging them to express their ideas, or preferences
- Negotiates a mutually agreed acceptable, safe, plan
- Open and honest about the result without being patronising
- Open and honest about the risks
- Avoids platitudes or false re-assurance

Communication with patients and their relatives

- Greets patient and obtains patient's name
- Introduces self, role
- Explains nature of interview (reason for coming to talk to patient)
- Assesses starting point: what patient understands already/is feeling
- Gives clear signposting that serious important information is to follow
- Chunks and checks, using patient's response to guide next steps

- Discovers what other information would help the patient, attempts to address patient's information needs
- Gives explanation in an organised manner (signposting/summarising)
- Uses clear language, avoids jargon and confusing language
- Picks up and responds to patient's non-verbal cues
- Allows patient time to react (use of silence, allows for shut-down)
- Recognises, acknowledges and validates patient's concerns and feelings (e.g. uses empathy)
- Appropriate non-verbal behaviour e.g. eye contact, posture and position, movement, facial expression, use of voice (pace, tone)
- Provides support: e.g. concern, understanding, willingness to help

Information gathering

- Obtains relevant history regarding her presenting symptoms and social history
- Obtains patients expectations and concerns

Applied clinical knowledge

- Demonstrates a sound and comprehensive evidence-based clinical knowledge
- Explanation of problem—(low grade cancer lining of the womb-staging not known)
- Investigations: MRI, chest x-ray for staging (spread)
- Hysterectomy with bilsateral salpingo-oophorectomy, may need pelvic lymph node dissection
- Explains total hysterectomy with bilateral salpingo-oophorectomy
- Usually stay in the hospital for two to three days with abdominal hysterectomy (one day if laparoscopic)

Further reading

Management of Endometrial Hyperplasia Green-top Guideline No. 67 RCOG/BSGE Joint Guideline | February 2016. https://www.rcog.org.uk/globalassets/documents/guidelines/green-top-guidelines/gtg_67_endometrial_hyperplasia.pdf

Task 6 **Lichen Sclerosus**

Instructions for Candidate

This task assesses the following clinical skills:

- Patient safety
- Communication with patients and their relatives
- Information gathering
- Applied clinical knowledge

Kirsten Hill is a 55-year-old fitness instructor.

She is having itching and soreness in her vulval area for many years. She thinks its candida and regularly uses over the counter antifungal preparations with no significant benefit. She feels that the itching is spreading around her back passage too.

She is married for 18 years and has three children. The itching is affecting her sex life and can disturb her sleep. She can't bear it any longer therefore contacted her GP.

When you examined her, the skin around the vulva and anus is shiny, white, and thin at places. It has the typical appearance of Lichen sclerosus.

You decide to go with this diagnosis.

Your task is to:

- Explain what lichen sclerosus is
- How can it be treated?
- What are the risks with Lichen sclerosus?

You have 10 minutes for this task (+ 2mins initial reading time).

Instructions for Assessor

Please read instructions to candidate and role player.

Record your overall clinical impression of the candidate for each domain (e.g. should this performance be pass, borderline, or a fail).

Instructions for Role Player

You are Kirsten Hill, 55-year-old fitness instructor.

The vulval itching has been brothering you for some years however you felt too embarrassed to seek help.

You had two children in the past both normal vaginal deliveries. You went through menopause two years ago.

You have been using over the counter antifungal preparations to control your symptoms but they haven't made much difference. You also keep the area very clean by washing it may times using soap and water.

You saw your GP as it's getting worse and affecting you sleep and relationship.

You are worried that you have some infection and will not be cured as nothing you are doing is helping.

You are also worried whether you have cancer as it bleeds sometimes after scratching.

Temperament: You are very annoyed and upset that why it's you. Why are the symptoms not improving although you are doing everything in your power?

Ideas: You are hoping that the treatment by the doctor will cure it all together

Concerns: You want to know long will it take to get rid of the condition. You want your life back. You are worried that you may give it to you husband.

Expectations: You want the doctor to explain what it is and what's the cause?
What the treatment involves and how long should she use it for?
Will it spread to the rest of your body?
What are the other complications? Can it turn into cancer?

Assessment

Marking Scheme

Patient safety:

Pass	Borderline	Fail

Communication with patients and their relatives:

Pass	Borderline	Fail

Information gathering:

Pass	Borderline	Fail

Applied clinical knowledge:

Pass	Borderline	Fail

Notes for Marking

Patient safety

- Assesses the patient's main concerns and ideas
- Discusses possible risks
- Involves patient in the process (e.g. encouraging them to express their ideas, or preferences)
- Open and honest about the risk of malignancy
- Explains long term chronic inflammatory condition with unknown etiology

Communication with patients and their relatives

- Greets, introduces self and role, checks patient's name
- Consent to proceed and explains nature of interview
- Assesses patient's starting point (what the patient wants to know) and sets the agenda
- Clear organised explanation in logical sequence
- Chunks: e.g. provides information in reasonable chunks
- Checks patient's understanding
- Language (easily understood, avoids or explains jargon)
- Uses visual aids appropriately e.g. diagrams or uses analogies to aid explanation

Information gathering

- Obtains relevant history regarding her vulval symptoms
- Obtains patients expectations and concerns

Applied clinical knowledge

- Demonstrates a sound and comprehensive evidence-based clinical knowledge
- Information about Lichen sclerosus is provided

Notes for Candidate

The scenario is taken from a common clinical scenario of our daily practice. It not only assesses the process of communication but also assesses the content of the knowledge given to the patient. It is important *how* you provide the information to the patient.

In counselling Ms Hill, the candidates must include the following:

- Lichen sclerosus is an inflammatory dermatosis that predominantly affects the anogenital area of women causing chronic vulval pruritus and dyspareunia. There is evidence that this is an autoimmune disease and that there is an increased incidence of tissue-specific antibodies and an increased association with other autoimmune diseases among patient.
- Two peak ages of presentation, the first of these occurs in prepubescent girls and the other is in post-menopausal women
- The true incidence is not known, but from referral patterns to vulval clinics the condition appears to be common
- The classical lesion is an ivory white, flat, polygonal, papule which on the vulva is usually confluent to produce plaques. The appearances of lichen sclerosus include pallor, atrophy, introital stenosis, burying of the clitoral hood and loss of architecture with central fusion. Purpuric lesions can often be found through local trauma. The vagina and cervix are not involved
- In the presence of vulval disease, extra genital lichen sclerosus is present in 11% of women, usually on the eyelids or on the back
- A vulval biopsy is not indicated, but should be considered if there are indurated or suspicious areas of skin. If the woman does not respond to treatment, then a biopsy should be considered
- There is an increased risk of squamous cell cancer of the vulva in women with lichen sclerosus The risk is small with a 5% figure often quoted but this likely to be lower as there are many women with undiagnosed LS (Lichen Sclerosus) in the community
- The management is topical potent corticosteroids e.g. 0.05% Clobetasol propionate ointment/ Dermovate on a reducing regimen
- Good skin care is essential and women must be advised to use emollients. They should use plain water to wash the perineal area and avoid soaps and bath salts
- Women with disease at the posterior fourchette can split during intercourse and this can lead to pain and sex avoidance. Women can use Dermovate massaged into the area of fissure and vaginal dilators can be suggested to patients to help overcome the introital narrowing and help treat vaginismus that might co-exist
- The treatment is life long and titrated according to her symptoms. Patient education is important, as is teaching the patient self-examination in order to detect potentially an early cancer

Practice this scenario with one of your friends who can act as a role player and ask another friend to provide you with feedback. We recommend you read the following:

Further reading

Powell JJ, Wojnarowska F. Lichen sclerosus. *Lancet*, 1999. 353: 1777–83.

Royal College of Obstetricians and Gynaecologist. The Management of Vulval Skin Disorders. Green-Top Guideline No. 58. London: RCOG; 2011. https://www.rcog.org.uk/globalassets/documents/guidelines/gtg_58.pdf

Chapter 19 **Urogynaecology and Pelvic Floor Problems**

Task 1 **Urodynamics**

Instructions for Candidate

This task assesses the following clinical skills:

- Patient safety
- Communication with patients and their relatives
- Information gathering
- Applied clinical knowledge

You are a ST5 doctor in the urogynaecology clinic. You are asked to see Amanda Scott, who is a 64-year-old woman. She has been referred by her GP with mixed urinary incontinence which has not responded to supervized pelvic floor muscle training, bladder retraining and Tolterodine. She is para 2 with two spontaneous vaginal deliveries. She has no significant medical or surgical history. Previous examination did not reveal any pelvic organ prolapse.

A urodynamic study was performed before her clinic appointment (see Fig 19.1). Amanda wishes to know more about the urodynamic findings and management options available to her. You will have ten minutes for the initial discussion. Once you have finished discussion with Amanda the assessor will ask you some questions.

You have 10 minutes for this task (+ 2mins initial reading time).

Instructions for Assessors

Please read instruction to candidate and actor.

There are some marks on the process mark sheet for the actor to assign at the end of the station.

Record your overall clinical impression of the candidate for each domain (i.e. should this performance be pass, borderline, or a fail).

Instructions for Role Player

You are Amanda Scott, a 64-year-old mother of two. You have been experiencing a sudden, desperate need to pass urine and urine leakage if you don't get to the toilet on time for the last three years. You also have episodes of unwanted loss of urine on coughing, laughing, physical exercise, and sexual intercourse.

Your bowel function is normal and you are not aware of any vaginal 'bulge'. You went through the 'change' (menopause) at the age of 52. You had two uneventful normal (vaginal) births. You are healthy without any previous operations.

You have seen a physiotherapist for pelvic floor exercises and you have tried a drug for your bladder called Tolterodine (one 2mg tablet twice a day). Unfortunately, you haven't seen any improvement of your symptoms.

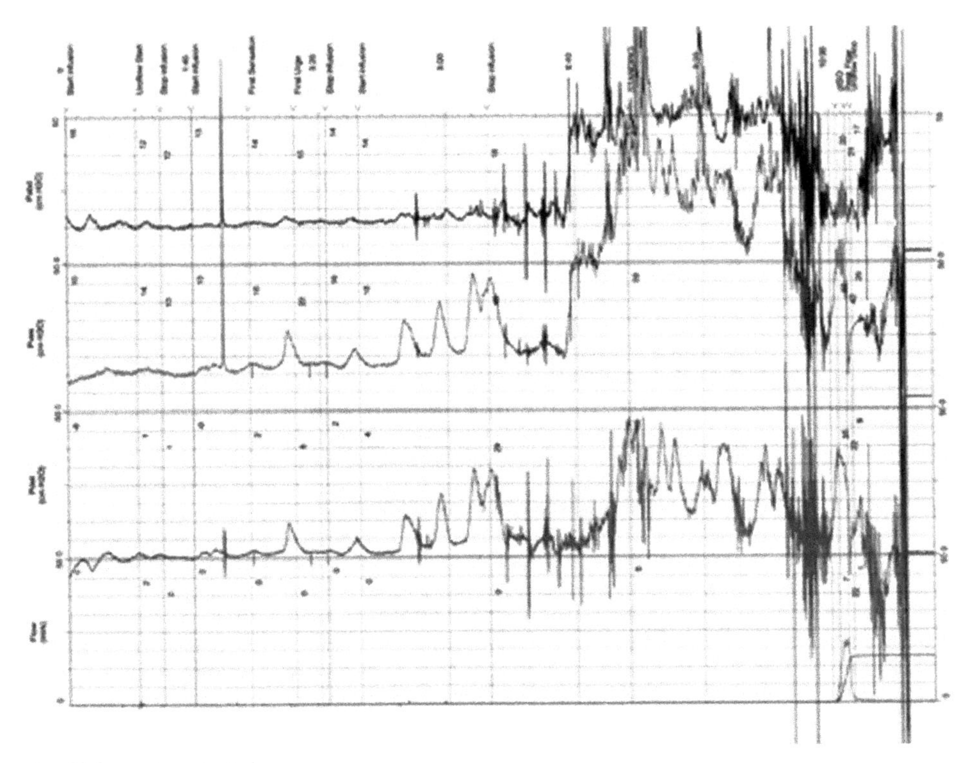

Fig. 19.1 Urodynamic study

Temperament: You think you are mostly a calm, level-headed woman, but you do like to be organized and in control of things. You find your symptoms very embarrassing.

Ideas: You are expecting a complete resolution of your symptoms as they impair your quality of life. You don't want to end up completely incontinent as your grandmother.

Concerns: You haven't seen any improvement with what you have tried so far. You are worried that you will need a catheter if there no other available options.

Expectations: You want the doctor to explain:

- What is the cause of your symptoms?
- What did the bladder function (urodynamic) test show?
- If there is need for further tests.
- What are your treatment options?
- The pros and cons of each treatment option

If the doctor doesn't mention it, please ask specifically for Botox injections in the bladder, the risk of needing a catheter after the operation and the need for repeat injections. Also ask if you could have surgery for your loss of urine on coughing, laughing, physical exercise

At the end there are some marks for you to award according to how well the candidate explained your questions and concerns.

Assessment

Marking Scheme

Patient safety:

Pass Borderline Fail

Communication with patients and their relatives:

Pass Borderline Fail

Information gathering:

Pass Borderline Fail

Applied clinical knowledge:

Pass Borderline Fail

Notes for Marking

Patient safety

- Assesses patient's main concerns and ideas
- Gives options and discusses the pros and cons of each
- Involves patient in the process (e.g. encouraging them to express their ideas, or preferences)
- Negotiates a mutually agreed, acceptable, and safe management plan

Communication with patients and their relatives

- Greets, introduces self and role, checks patient's name
- Assesses patient's starting point (what the patient wants to know) and sets the agenda
- Clear organised explanation in logical sequence
- Chunks: i.e. provides information in reasonable chunks
- Checks patient's understanding
- Language (easily understood, avoids or explains jargon)
- Uses visual aids appropriately e.g. diagrams or uses analogies to aid explanation
- Honest about complications associated with intravesical botox

Information gathering

- Obtains a relevant urogynaecology history
- Obtains patient's views, expectations, and concerns

Applied clinical knowledge

- Demonstrates a sound and comprehensive evidence-based clinical knowledge
- Counsels the patient with relevant information that is factually correct
- Makes a robust and safe management plan

Notes for Candidate

Explanation of urodynamic findings

- Spontaneous and provoked detrusor overactivity
- Unable to assess for urodynamic stress incontinence as persistent involuntary detrusor contractions
- No voiding dysfunction (reassuring pressure-flow study)

Cause of symptoms

- Idiopathic in most of the cases, unless neurological abnormality
- Not associated with prolapse in her case

Need for further investigations

- Consider cystoscopy in refractory cases

Management options

- Alternative antimuscarinic drugs. Consider extended modified release agents (Tolterodine, Oxybutynin etc) or selective agents (Darifenacin, Solifenacin)
- Mirabegron (beta-3 adrenoceptor agonist). Better safety profile, no antimuscarinic side effects
- Botulinum toxin A. Explain risk of UTI, risk of voiding difficulties requiring CISC and need for repeat injections every six to 12 months
- Posterior Tibial Nerve Stimulation. Explain need to attend every week for 12 weeks and then 'top-ups' every four to 12 weeks depending on the symptoms
- Sacral Nerve Stimulation. Insertion of electrical stimulator in sacral area only in tertiary referral centres
- Need to control urgency before considering surgery for stress urinary incontinence

Further reading

Urinary Incontinence in women—management CG 171Last updated 2015. https://www.nice.org.uk/guidance/cg171?unlid=6517475942016319221354

Task 2 **Prolapse**

Instructions for Candidate

This task assesses the following clinical skills:

- Patient safety
- Communication with patients and their relatives
- Information gathering
- Applied clinical knowledge

You are an ST5 doctor in the gynaecology clinic with your consultant. Your consultant has asked you to take a brief history from Barbara Smith who is a 67-year-old retired nurse. Please take a brief history. You do not need to examine her. Once you have taken the history, you will be asked to give a brief summary with relevant points to the assessor.

You will be provided with examination findings and asked some questions by the assessor.

You have 10 minutes for this task (+ 2mins initial reading time).

Instructions for Assessors

Please read instructions to candidate and actor.

Allow the candidate to conduct the interview undisturbed unless they are straying off the track of the question (in which case you can show them their instructions again)

The patient has symptoms of prolapse. The history should cover:

- Extent, duration and degree of inconvenience
- Associated bladder symptoms—frequency, urgency, urgency incontinence, stress incontinence, urinary tract infections, or voiding dysfunction
- Any bowel problems including need for digitation
- Any interference with sexual life
- Medical, surgical and family history
- Daily intake—output
- Whether referred to the physiotherapist/continence advisory service
- Any management undertaken in primary care

Once the candidate has taken a relevant history and presented to you, provide the candidate with the following information:

- BMI—29
- Abdominal examination—unremarkable
- Vaginal examination—vault prolapse stage III
- Bimanual examination—no masses felt
- Atrophic vagina

Now ask the candidate to explain the examination findings and discuss the standard common options of management including surgical management to Mrs Smith.

There are some marks on the process mark sheet for the actor to assign at the end of the station. Record your overall clinical impression of the candidate for each domain (e.g. should this be pass, borderline, or a fail).

Instructions for Role Player

You are Barbara Smith, retired nurse, aged 67 years. You are married for 45 years to Steve. You have got two children age 42 and 39 years, both delivered normally. You have had an abdominal hysterectomy (hysterectomy through your tummy) along with removal your tubes and ovaries for very heavy periods and fibroids at the age of 48 years. You have been reasonably well since. Recently you have felt and noticed a lump coming down in your vagina. This is quite bothersome and interfering with your sexual life. You do not have much problem with your bladder other than needing to go to the toilet quite frequently (frequency), taking a while to initiate the flow and sometimes you do not feel like the bladder has emptied completely. Your bowels are normal. You GP has examined you and said you have got a 'prolapse'.

If you are specifically asked:

- You have not had any water infections
- You do not have to push the lump up to empty your bowels
- You have to lean forward to empty your bladder and sometimes dribble afterwards
- The GP tried something called a ring pessary which came out after 24 hours
- You never had any other treatments for the prolapse
- You were not referred to physiotherapists or continence nurses
- You have no medical issues other than high blood pressure which is controlled with tablets
- You drink five cups of coffee and a litre of water daily
- You are a non-smoker and drink alcohol socially

Concerns: You are very concerned about what prolapse actually means and its implications on your life. You are quite bothered with this lump interfering with your life.

Expectation: Keen to sort the problem to be able to have a normal active life. You do not want to try another pessary and looking forward to being offered an alternative solution or an operation.

Assessment

Marking Scheme

Patient safety:

Pass	Borderline	Fail

Communication with patients and their relatives:

Pass	Borderline	Fail

Information gathering:

Pass	Borderline	Fail

Applied clinical knowledge:

Pass	Borderline	Fail

Notes for Marking

Patient safety

- Assesses patients main concern and ideas
- Gives options and discusses pros and cons

- Discusses possible complications
- Involves patient in the process (e.g. encouraging them to express their ideas and preferences)
- Negotiates a mutually agreed safe acceptable plan
- Open and honest about giving information
- Manage patient expectations and give a clear idea of the desired outcome of a successful operation
- Being honest about the complications associated with surgery specially risk of recurrence, re-operation rate and patient satisfaction
- Provides information about surgeon performing the procedure e.g. competent and trained surgeon or junior doctor under direct supervision
- Need for discussion at multidisciplinary meeting

Communication with patients and their relatives

- Greets, introduces self and role, checks patients name
- Consent to proceed and explains nature of the interview
- Assesses patient's starting point (what patient wants to know) and sets the agenda
- Clear and organised explanation in logical sequence
- Chunks: e.g. provides information in reasonable chunks
- Checks patient understanding
- Language (easily understood, avoids and explains jargon)
- Uses visual aids appropriately e.g. diagrams or uses analogies to aid explanation
- Written information provided appropriately
- Presents a clear and succinct history to assessor

Information gathering

- Obtains a relevant urogynaecology history
- Obtains patient's views, expectations, and concerns

Application of knowledge

- Demonstrates comprehensive evidence-based clinical knowledge
- Obtains a comprehensive history including impact on quality of life
- Discusses all options of management plan including no intervention, trial of another pessary, pelvic floor muscle training, vaginal oestrogens and surgery
- Explains the pros and cons of abdominal/laparoscopic sacrocolpopexy vs sacrospinous fixation

Notes for Candidate

This scenario is a common clinical presentation in gynaecology or urogynaecology clinics in our daily practice. It not only assesses the process of communication and communication skills but also assesses the content of the clinical knowledge and information given to the patient. It is important you get the salient points in the history and determine patient's main concern and the fact that she is keen for an operation. It is also important how you provide the information and what information you provide.

The history should cover:

- Extent, duration and degree of inconvenience
- Associated bladder symptoms—frequency, urgency, urgency incontinence, stress incontinence, urinary tract infections, or voiding dysfunction
- Any bowel problems including need for digitation

- Any interference with sexual life
- Medical, surgical and family history
- Daily intake—output
- Whether referred to the physiotherapist/continence advisory service
- Any management undertaken in primary care

You should discuss the common surgical procedures available along with the positives and negative aspects of abdominal sacrocolpopexy (ASC) and sacrospinous fixation (SSF):

- Route of both procedures; ASC can be done laparoscopically
- Method of vault fixation
- Both effective treatment
- Recurrence rate
- Re-operation rate, patient reported symptoms, objective failure at any site and patient satisfaction similar with both procedures
- ASC associated with significantly lower rates of recurrent vault prolapse, dyspareunia and post-operative stress urinary incontinence (SUI) compared to SSF
- SSF associated with earlier recovery and return to work, less operating time
- ASC not appropriate in women with complex/multiple abdominal surgery
- SSF not appropriate in women with short vagina and with a history of dyspareunia
- Other complications with ASC—bowel injury, sacral myelitis, severe bleeding, mesh erosion
- Other complications with SSF—buttock pain, post-operative anterior compartment prolapse and SUI, pudendal nerve injury, irritation of sciatic nerve, partial ureteral obstruction
- Follow up with patient reported outcome including success rate, relief of presenting symptoms and objective cure rate
- Surgery is undertaken by experienced surgeon with required training or performed by trainees under direct supervision
- Clinicians work as part of MDT and case discussed in MDT meeting
- Patient information leaflets to be given

Further reading

Post Hysterectomy Vaginal Vault Prolapse; Green-top guideline No 46; RCOG/BSUG Joint Guideline; July 2015. https://www.rcog.org.uk/globalassets/documents/guidelines/gtg-46.pdf

Task 3 **Incontinence: stress urinary incontinence**

Instructions for Candidate

This task assesses the following clinical skills:

- Patient safety
- Communication with patients and their relatives
- Information gathering
- Applied clinical knowledge

You are the ST5 in the gynaecology clinic; your next patient is a Mrs Mills, referred to you by her GP due to 'stress incontinence'.

Your task is to:

- Take a full history from her (you do not need to examine her- examination findings will be given to you by the assessor)
- Explain the different treatment options
- Answer any of her questions

You have 10 minutes for this task (+ 2mins initial reading time).

Instructions for Assessors

Please read instruction to candidate and actor.

Allow the candidate to conduct the interview undisturbed unless they are straying off the track of the question (in which case you can show them their instructions again).

This patient has stress incontinence, the history of presenting complaint should cover:

- The extent, duration and inconvenience caused by the symptoms
- Obstetric history—number of children, mode of delivery, birth weights
- Urinary history—assess for signs of urgency
- Sexual history e.g. leaking during intercourse
- Smoking history
- Any pelvic floor exercises done
- Smear history
- Family planning issues
- Past medical and surgical history
- Family history, social history, and current drug history

Once the candidate has taken a relevant history and presented to you, provide the candidate with following information:

Abdominal examination—unremarkable
Speculum examination—cervix satisfactory
Bimanual examination—normal sized, mobile, anteverted uterus, no adnexal masses or tenderness, demonstrable stress incontinence on three coughs

Now ask the candidate to explain the management plan to Mrs Mills. The management plan should emphasize the need for supervized pelvic floor muscle treatment.

There are some marks on the process mark sheet for the actor to assign at the end of the station.

Record your overall clinical impression of the candidate for each domain (i.e. should this performance be pass, borderline, or a fail).

Instructions for Role Player

You are Mrs Mills, a 35-year-old woman who had her first child two years ago by forceps delivery. Since then you have suffered from incontinence problems. Recently you caught your son's cold and found that you leaked urine when you coughed a lot.

Your son has become very active running around and wants you to join in. You find it difficult to run after him or go on the trampoline as you are nervous about leaking urine.

You and your partner are unsure about whether you want more children. You had always thought you wanted two children but your partner is unsure about it due to financial reasons.

You want to know what your options are to help resolve this problem as you can't believe you are so young and yet are unable to run around anymore. You don't want to have any treatment that may affect your ability to have children in the future. You are worried that without help you won't be able to do even simple things like walking, without leaking.

You smoke ten cigarettes a day and have not been able to lose the weight you put on in pregnancy—you now have a BMI of 30. You remember being taught pelvic floor exercises at your antenatal classes, and do them when you can remember.

Temperament: You think you are a calm, level headed woman although you are very anxious about this problem.

Ideas: You are expecting there to be a quick fix solution to your problem. You are not ready to decide to future children now.

Concerns: you are concerned that this will get worse. You remember your grandmother wearing nappies and are concerned this will happen to you.

Expectations: You want the doctor to explain the following:

How to improve things?
How common this is?
What will happen if you have more children?

Assessment

Marking Scheme

Patient safety:
Pass Borderline Fail

Communication with patients and their relatives:
Pass Borderline Fail

Information gathering:
Pass Borderline Fail

Applied clinical knowledge:
Pass Borderline Fail

Notes for marking

Patient safety

- Assesses the patient's main concerns and ideas
- Gives options and discusses the pros and cons of different management plans
- Discusses possible complications and measures to reduce them
- Involves patient in the process (e.g. encouraging them to express their ideas, or preferences)
- Negotiates a mutually agreed acceptable, safe, plan
- Open and honest about options and possible complications and natural history of stress incontinence
- Explain mechanism in place to deal with complications and learn from such complication

Communication with patients and their relatives

- Greets, introduces self and role, checks patient's name
- Consent to proceed and explains nature of interview
- Assesses patient's starting point (what the patient wants to know) and sets the agenda
- Clear organised explanation in logical sequence
- Chunks: i.e. provides information in reasonable chunks
- Checks patient's understanding.
- Language (easily understood, avoids or explains jargon)

Information gathering

- Obtains a relevant urogynaecology history
- Obtains patient's views, expectations, and concerns

Applied clinical knowledge

- Demonstrates a sound and comprehensive evidencebased clinical knowledge
- Explains the need for supervised pelvic floor muscle treatment
- Encourages to lose weight and offers lifestyle advice
- Uses visual aids appropriately e.g. diagrams or uses analogies to aid explanation
- Presents a clear and succinct history to the assessor

Further reading

Urinary Incontinence in women—management CG 171Last updated 2015. https://www.nice.org.uk/guidance/cg171?unlid=6517475942016319221354

Task 4 **Incontinence—stress urinary incontinence**

Instructions for Candidate

This task assesses the following clinical skills:

- Patient safety
- Communication with patients and their relatives
- Information gathering
- Applied clinical knowledge

You are the ST5 in the gynaecology clinic; your next patient is a Mrs Spencer, referred to you by her GP due to a long standing history of 'stress incontinence'.

Your task is to:

- Take a full history from her (you do not need to examine her- examination findings will be given to you by the assessor)
- Explain the different treatment options
- Answer any of her questions

You have 10 minutes for this task (+ 2mins initial reading time).

Instructions for Assessors

Please read instruction to candidate and actor.

Allow the candidate to conduct the interview undisturbed unless they are straying off the track of the question (in which case you can show them their instructions again).

This patient has stress incontinence, the history of presenting complaint should cover:

- The extent, duration and inconvenience caused by the symptoms
- Obstetric history—number of children, mode of delivery, birth weights
- Urinary history—assess for signs of urgency
- Sexual history e.g. leaking during intercourse
- Smoking history
- Any pelvic floor exercises done
- Smear history
- Family planning issues
- Past medical and surgical history
- Family history, social history, and current drug history

Once the candidate has taken a relevant history and presented to you, provide the candidate with following information:

Abdominal examination—unremarkable
Speculum examination—cervix satisfactory
Bimanual examination—normal sized, mobile, anteverted uterus, no adnexal masses or tenderness, demonstrable stress incontinence on three coughs

Now ask the candidate to explain the management plan to Mrs Spencer.

There are some marks on the process mark sheet for the actor to assign at the end of the station.

Record your overall clinical impression of the candidate for each domain (i.e. should this performance be pass, borderline, or a fail).

Instructions for Role Player

You are Mrs Spencer, a 62-year-old woman who has suffered from incontinence problems for the last ten years.

You have seen doctors in the past for this, have seen physiotherapists and tried very conscientiously with your pelvic floor exercises. However you have seen little to no improvement in your symptoms.

You need to wear pads all the time and want surgery to end this problem once and for all. You feel you have tried everything else—you have lost a lot of weight, sorted out your constipation issues, but nothing has helped.

Temperament: You think you are a calm, level headed woman who can take in information rationally.

Ideas: You have read some information on the internet and very much want surgical management now.

Concerns: you are concerned that this will get worse if surgery isn't offered.

Expectations: You want to be offered surgical management.

You want the doctor to explain the following:

Risks of surgery?
Success rates?
Recovery time?
Length of stay in hospital?

Assessment

Marking Scheme

Patient safety:

Pass	Borderline	Fail

Communication with patients and their relatives:

Pass	Borderline	Fail

Information gathering:

Pass	Borderline	Fail

Applied clinical knowledge:

Pass	Borderline	Fail

Notes for Marking

Patient safety

- Assesses the patient's main concerns and ideas
- Gives options and discusses the pros and cons of different management plans
- Discusses possible complications and measures to reduce them
- Involves patient in the process (e.g. encouraging them to express their ideas or preferences
- Negotiates a mutually agreed acceptable, safe plan
- Open and honest about procedure and possible complications

- Provides patient with information about the person performing the procedure and safeguard in place i.e. competent clinician or junior doctor under direct supervision. Explains mechanism in place to deal with complications and learn from complications. Is honest about prolongation of recovery time if untoward complication happen

Communication with patients and their relatives

- Greets, introduces self and role, checks patient's name
- Consent to proceed and explains nature of interview
- Assesses patient's starting point (what the patient wants to know) and sets the agenda
- Clear organised explanation in logical sequence
- Chunks: i.e. provides information in reasonable chunks
- Checks patient's understanding.
- Language (easily understood, avoids or explains jargon)
- Uses visual aids appropriately e.g. diagrams or uses analogies to aid explanation
- Presents a clear and succinct history to the assessor

Information gathering

- Obtains a relevant urogynaecology history
- Obtains patient's views, expectations and concerns

Applied clinical knowledge

- Demonstrates a sound and comprehensive evidencebased clinical knowledge
- Elicits salient points in the history e.g. effect of incontinence on quality of life
- Discusses various surgical options i.e. midurethral tape, injectables, colposuspension
- Explains briefly about advantages and disadvantages of each procedure

Further reading

Urinary Incontinence in women—management CG 171Last updated 2015. https://www.nice.org.uk/guidance/cg171?unlid=6517475942016319221354

Task 5 **Midurethral tape**

Instructions for Candidate

This task assesses the following clinical skills:

- Patient safety
- Communication with patients and their relatives
- Information gathering
- Applied clinical knowledge

You are the ST5 in the gynaecology clinic and your consultant has asked you to see Mrs Johns who needs to be consented for a midurethral tape procedure.

Your task is to:

- Explain the procedure to her
- Explain the associated risks and complications
- Answer any of her questions

You have 10 minutes for this task (+ 2mins initial reading time).

Instruction to Assessors

Please read instruction to candidate and role player.

Allow the candidate to conduct the interview undisturbed unless they are straying off the track of the question (in which case you can show them their instructions again).

There are some marks on the process mark sheet for the actor to assign at the end of the station.

Record your overall clinical impression of the candidate for each domain (i.e. should this performance be pass, borderline, or a fail).

Instructions to Role Player

You are Mrs Johns a 55-year-old woman who has been suffering from urinary incontinence for the past ten years. It has been becoming increasingly bad over the last few years and is now affecting your quality of life significantly. You have stopped being able to go your aerobics class for fear of leaking and have therefore stopped exercising which is not helping you to try and lose weight.

You have had two children born by forceps delivery. You are otherwise fit and well, apart from being overweight.

You understand that a "mesh" will be used in the operation and so have done some research online and read some concerning reports about mesh erosion. You have been very alarmed by what you have read and are now not sure that you wish to go ahead with the operation. You have read that it has ruined many women's lives and have concerns about the mesh going into the bladder and not being able to have it removed.

Temperament: You think you are a calm, level headed woman although you are very anxious about this problem and complications from surgery.

Ideas: You are expecting there to be a quick fix solution to your problem. You want there to be a guarantee that things won't go wrong.

Concerns: You are concerned that you will end up like the people you have read about on the internet, being worse off after the operation than you were before.

Expectations: You want the doctor to explain the following:

What the success rates are?
What the complication rates are?
How soon can you go home?
What happens if something goes wrong?

Assessment

Marking Scheme

Patient safety:
Pass Borderline Fail

Communication with patients and their relatives:
Pass Borderline Fail

Information gathering:
Pass Borderline Fail

Applied clinical knowledge:
Pass Borderline Fail

Notes for Marking

Patient safety

- Assesses the patient's main concerns and ideas
- Gives options and discusses the pros and cons of surgical management
- Discusses possible complications and measures to reduce them
- Involves patient in the process (e.g. encouraging them to express their ideas, or preferences)
- Negotiates a mutually agreed acceptable, safe, plan
- Open and honest about options and possible complications of surgical management
- Explain mechanism in place to deal with complications and learn from such complication
- Provides patient with information about the person performing the procedure and safeguard in place i.e. competent clinician or junior doctor under direct supervision
- Being honest about prolongation of recovery time if untoward complications happen

Communication with patients and their relatives

- Greets, introduces self and role, checks patient's name
- Consent to proceed and explains nature of interview
- Assesses patient's starting point (what the patient wants to know) and sets the agenda
- Clear organised explanation in logical sequence
- Chunks: i.e. provides information in reasonable chunks
- Checks patient's understanding
- Language (easily understood, avoids or explains jargon)
- Uses visual aids appropriately e.g. diagrams or uses analogies to aid explanation

Information gathering

- Obtains a relevant urogynaecology history
- Obtains patient's views, expectations, and concerns

Applied clinical knowledge

- Demonstrates a sound and comprehensive evidence-based clinical knowledge
- Ensures conservative treatment has been tried
- Small volume of mesh is used
- Small risk of erosion exists
- Efficacy data of retropubic midurethral tapes exists over 18 years
- Discusses alternative method like colposuspension, injectables

Further reading

Urinary Incontinence in women—management CG 171. Last updated 2015. https://www.nice.org.uk/guidance/cg171?unlid=6517475942016319221354

Chapter 20 **Developing Professionalism**

Task 1 **Difficult patient**

Instructions for Candidate

This task assesses the following clinical skills:

- Patient safety
- Communication with patients and their relatives
- Information gathering
- Applied clinical knowledge

You are in the antenatal clinic and are about to see Kelly Morgan, a 23-year-old nulliparous patient. She is 37 + 3 and this is her first pregnancy. She has been classified as low risk, and has been under midwifery care until now. Her community midwife has sent her to the clinic because she has been requesting induction of labour because she is exhausted and 'unable to cope'. There have been no concerns about foetal growth or movements, her blood pressure and urinalysis are normal, and she has no medical co-morbidities. She had a normal ultrasound scan at 36 weeks. The clinic is running over an hour late as your consultant is off sick. You have been told by the clinic staff that she has already been complaining about the delay.

The hospital has a very definite policy against induction of labour for non-obstetric reasons. Your task is to explore Kelly's concerns and to explain to her that her request for IOL is not something that is usually done in this context.

You have 10 minutes for this task (+ 2mins initial reading time).

Instructions for Assessor

This clinical assessment task assesses the candidate's ability to professionally deal with an angry patient. This needs robust communication skills to defuse the situation at the same time exploring the patient's concerns and making a safe plan. Please do not interrupt or prompt the candidate.

Please mark each domain as pass, borderline, or fail.

Instruction for Role Player

At this station, you are very angry and upset.

You are Kelly Morgan, a 23-year-old admin assistant. This is your first pregnancy, and you have found it difficult from the very beginning. You had morning sickness until 18 weeks, and ever since 30 weeks you have felt absolutely exhausted. You have no energy, your back hurts and you just want this baby delivered. Your midwives keep telling you that this is all normal, and that it's better to wait for natural labour, but you don't care if you end up with a caesarean section. You are fed up with being fobbed off by people who don't know what they are talking about. You want to complain because no-one is listening to you. You are also worried because your best friend had a stillbirth at 38 weeks and can't stop thinking about whether the same thing will happen to you (do not disclose this unless the candidate asks if there is anything particular that you are worried about). Your partner works all the time and you are feeling really unsupported.

Assessment

Marking scheme		
Patient safety:		
Pass	Borderline	Fail
Communication with patients and their relatives:		
Pass	Borderline	Fail
Information gathering:		
Pass	Borderline	Fail
Applied clinical knowledge:		
Pass	Borderline	Fail

Notes for Marking

Patient safety

- Reassurance—36 week scan normal, measurements normal, foetal movements normal
- Asks about support at home
- Offers further appointment for reassurance; offers second opinion from consultant
- Apologizes for the clinic running late

Communication with patients and their relatives

- Greeting, introduction, good eye contact
- Sympathetic approach- non aggressive response
- Speaks in a calm manner, appropriate volume
- Attentive listening to patient's concerns
- Acknowledges patient's feelings and displays empathy
- Makes attempt to defuse anger of patient
- Acknowledges patient's wish to complain and signposts to complaints procedure

Information gathering

- Asks about why patient wants to be induced- elicits history of back pain and tiredness
- Explores other underlying worries—elicits history of stillbirth in best friend

Applied clinical knowledge

- Explains risks of induction of labour-more painful, longer labour, failed induction
- Explains recommendation to not induce unless medical reasons
- Discusses managing back pain- analgesia, mobility, physiotherapy, etc.

Notes for Candidate

The core skills and knowledge that are tested under this module in the RCOG training curriculum are broad based and applicable to all scenarios that you might come across both in the examination and in real life. It is important to demonstrate that as well as the knowledge and skills, you also have the professionalism to work effectively with your patients and colleagues. Important facets of professionalism include communication, team working, leadership, negotiation and diplomacy. These skills are essential to have when working as an independent practitioner, and will often form part of the marking scheme in a clinical assessment task.

The difficult patient

This is one of the clinical assessment task that is most feared by candidates as it tests their ability to communicate effectively with a patient, who will have been briefed to make the encounter difficult. Losing control of the situation and allowing it to escalate can mean that you lose your opportunity to score marks as the scenario unfolds. It is therefore important to remain professional and maintain control. The 'difficult' patient encompasses a wide variety of different situations, which can be challenging for the doctor, patient, or often both. Most difficult patient encounters have a multitude of factors that contribute towards the problem. Patients can be un-cooperative, hostile, demanding and unpleasant, or they may have unrealistic expectations of their doctor or their treatment. Often the patient's underlying condition can be a factor in making interactions more challenging. Conditions such as chronic pelvic pain are inherently more difficult to manage, and this can lead to frustrating encounters for both the doctor and patient.

The most important thing to remember when approaching a station with a difficult patient is to remain calm. Don't allow your anxiety about the encounter to be revealed in your manner, voice or body language. Be aware of your body language and avoid closed positions, such as arms crossed. Allow the patient to talk and verbalize their concerns and issues- avoid arguing with them or talking over them, as this can escalate the situation. Demonstrating that you are listening, by acknowledging what the patient is saying, nodding as they talk, and echoing their words back to them, will show that you are an empathetic doctor who is taking their concerns seriously. An early step that can help to defuse the situation is to acknowledge that you are in the midst of a difficult conversation, for example saying, 'I can see you are very upset about what has happened, so we are both finding this conversation quite difficult. Would you agree with that?' This encourages the patient to engage with you in moving forward, rather than continuing to dwell on their anger or upset. Try and see the consultation from the patient's perspective.

Most patients are not difficult for no reason. There will usually be underlying factors that are contributing towards their behaviour, such as anxiety about their own condition, worry about a loved one (e.g. their baby in an obstetric scenario), or personal/financial concerns related to their health. Exploring this or acknowledging this will make the patient feel more supported, and will hopefully help them see that you understand their problems. If the scenario involves something that has gone wrong with their care, make sure you apologize (for more on this type of scenario, see Task 2).

Once you have brought the situation under control, then you can focus on moving the situation forward and finding a solution to whatever the problem is, or at the very least, a plan for how to proceed. Ensure that the patient knows that you understand their concerns and that you want to help them. Talk to the patient, repeat back to them what you perceive the problem to be, and outline your plan for how to move forward or possible treatment solutions if applicable. As always, at the end ask the patient if they have any questions or if there is anything else they would like to say to you.

Most clinical assessment tasks focusing on the difficult patient will involve angry or upset patients. A more difficult situation is the patient who talks too much during a history taking station. Role players may have been briefed to keep talking and giving irrelevant, tangential details that are unrelated to the clinical scenario. This can be a challenge as it makes it difficult for you to focus on the areas where you will glean information and score points. This is a test of your ability to effectively steer a clinical encounter. You shouldn't be rude to the patient, e.g. by talking over her. The most useful approach is to say, 'I'm very sorry to interrupt, but we unfortunately only have limited time. Would you mind if we went back to … … …?' Then get back on track and ask your next question. It's acceptable to do this several times if you need to. Ensure that you smile and keep your overall manner pleasant, and the patient should respond appropriately to your request.

Further reading

Dealing with angry and aggressive patients, Karthik Vishwanathan,12 Aug 2006, BMJ careers. http://careers.bmj.com/careers/advice/view-article.html?id=1854#

Task 2 **Colleague in difficulty**

Instruction for Candidate

This task assesses the following clinical skills:

- Patient safety
- Communication with patients and their relatives
- Information gathering
- Applied clinical knowledge

You have been called to see Jennifer Mullins on the surgical high dependency unit. She is a 36 year-old-who was seen in the early pregnancy unit yesterday with minimal PV bleeding at six weeks' gestation. A diagnosis of a missed miscarriage was made on ultrasound. After counselling, she opted for surgical management of miscarriage, which was carried out this morning by one of your colleagues who has now left to go to a clinic at a peripheral hospital. She has a history of two previous caesarean sections and a uterine rupture in her last pregnancy and so the registrar who booked her for the surgery suggested that the procedure be done under ultrasound guidance. For reasons unknown, this advice was not followed and the procedure was done blindly. During the procedure, bleeding was noted and a uterine perforation was suspected. A laparoscopy was undertaken, and this showed a uterine perforation. Unfortunately, a small bowel injury was also found—she went on to have a laparotomy and primary repair of the small bowel.

Your consultant is busy with a complex emergency in theatre, and the ward has asked you to come and explain to the patient what has happened, as she is becoming increasingly anxious.

You have 10 minutes for this task (+ 2mins initial reading time).

Instructions for Assessor

This clinical assessment task assesses the candidate's ability to perform duty of candour and explain factually the sequence of events leading up to the complication

Please do not interrupt or prompt the candidate.

Please mark each domain as pass, borderline, or fail.

Instructions for Role Player

You are Jennifer Mullins, a 36-year-old teacher. You already have two children. This pregnancy was a planned pregnancy with your new partner, and you were devastated to be told that you had miscarried. You were offered various options for how to treat this miscarriage, and opted to have an operation as you wanted it over and done with. You were worried about the uterine rupture that you had in your last pregnancy, and specifically asked if anything could be done to reduce the risk of more damage to your uterus during the procedure. You were reassured that the surgeon would use an ultrasound machine to reduce this risk. You have woken up in the surgical HDU connected to lots of monitors, with a catheter in and with a big dressing on your abdomen. You are very scared and upset, and want to know what has happened.

Questions you may ask:

- Why did this happen?
- Didn't the surgeon use the ultrasound machine?
- Did I have to have a hysterectomy?
- Will I be able to get pregnant again?

- Is this because a junior doctor operated on me? Why didn't the consultant operate on me?
- Does this mean I have to poo into a bag? Am I going to be incontinent in the future?

Assessment

Marking Scheme

Patient safety:
Pass Borderline Fail

Communication with patients and their relatives:
Pass Borderline Fail

Information gathering:
Pass Borderline Fail

Applied clinical knowledge:
Pass Borderline Fail

Notes for Marking

Patient safety

- Addressing the patient's other concerns
- Procedure was carried out by an individual who has been trained and is competent in this procedure
- Future fertility should not be affected
- Colostomy was not done; no association with bowel incontinence
- Acknowledges that patient is upset, offers support
- Offers general reassurance, i.e. injury repaired, on HDU for monitoring, expected to recover well etc.
- Duty of Candour
- Is open, honest and non-defensive
- Apologizes for complication
- Explains that there will be an investigation into whether the complication could have been prevented
- Explains that patient will be told outcome of this investigation
- Explains that will be given contact details for someone to contact regarding the investigation
- Explains that plan to use ultrasound guidance was not followed, and that this could be a relevant factor

Communication with patients and their relatives

- Greeting, introduction, good eye contact
- Sympathetic approach
- Speaks in a calm manner, appropriate volume
- Attentive listening to patient's concerns
- Acknowledges patient's feelings and displays empathy
- Acknowledges patient is scared and upset

Information gathering

- Obtains relevant information surrounding the procedure
- Obtains patients views, expectations, and concerns

Applied clinical knowledge

- Explains what happened during the procedure
- During the course of evacuation, bleeding was seen and this raised the possibility of injury to the uterus
- Therefore a laparoscopy was carried out (keyhole) to look at any damage, and this confirmed perforation
- A hole in the bowel was also seen, which is why a larger incision had to be done on the abdomen
- The bowel was repaired, without the need for a colostomy
- Acknowledges that the patient's previous history may have contributed to this.

Notes for Candidate

Team work

Team work is integral to practice in obstetrics and gynaecology, and any number of scenarios may require you to make reference to team working, for example multidisciplinary team working in gynaecological oncology. The General Medical Council's *Good Medical Practice* states that 'You must work collaboratively with colleagues, respecting their skills and contributions; you must treat colleagues fairly and with respect; you must be aware of how your behaviour may influence others within and outside of the team'.

In an emergency skills station, it will be important to state to the examiner that you will summon the help of the rest of the team, for example the midwife in charge, the anaesthetist, the neonatologist, etc. In other scenarios, it is advized to simply stop and think of whether your assessment, treatment or overall approach would be enhanced by having another team member present. If the answer is yes, then say so.

Colleague in difficulty

Doctors may get into difficulties for a number of reasons, including poor health, family problems, overwork and burnout, or professional isolation. Addressing and acting on these concerns may be very stressful and difficult when they relate to a colleague with whom you work closely, or if that colleague is senior to you. However if an individual's behaviour poses a risk to the safety of patients, colleagues or the public, or if it constitutes unacceptable conduct (e.g. criminal behaviour), then is important for this to be acted upon. The GMC's Good Medical Practice guidance states clearly that 'Doctors must protect patients from risk of risk of harm posed by a colleagues' conduct, performance or health'.

Significant concerns about a doctor's performance may arise secondary to a number of different situations. Examples that may come up in a clinical assessment task include poor clinical performance, concerns over alcohol or drug use, bullying or harassment of staff or patients, health problems leading to poor practice, poor administration leading to an effect on patient care, or poor team working and leadership.

The most important factor to remember when addressing a scenario like this is to keep patient safety as the main priority. If the individual is in situation where there is an immediate threat to patient safety (e.g. suspected of being under the influence of alcohol whilst in theatre- a 'classic' clinical assessment task scenario), then immediate action must be taken to remove them from that situation. Alongside this principle, it is also important to demonstrate care and compassion for your colleague.

The National Patient Safety Agency has issued written advice on what to do if you have concerns about a colleague's performance. These principles are a useful framework for approaching this type of situation. Healthcare organizations should have a policy covering how to raise a concern, and this should be followed. The first point of contact is usually your 'line manager', who in practical terms will be the clinical director of your department, or perhaps your educational supervisor. The person with ultimate responsibility for issues such as this will be the medical director of the hospital. It is important that you do not say that you will investigate any concerns that you might have yourself, as this could constitute misconduct on your part. The person who is named by the organization as being responsible for investigating this type of concern will usually make contact with the clinician involved and tell them that a concern has been raised about their performance or conduct. The identity of the person who has raised the concern will normally remain confidential, unless there are reasons related to any investigation or legal process which require it to be disclosed.

Equality and diversity

Equality is defined as ensuring that individuals or groups of individuals are treated fairly and equally and no less favourably regardless of their race, gender, disability, religion (or other beliefs), sexual orientation, age, etc. Promotion of equality in healthcare aims to ensure that there is no discrimination in terms of access to healthcare or treatment. Diversity aims to recognize, respect and value the differences between individuals, and to promote inclusivity.

In the UK, the relevant legislation is The Equality Act 2010, which allows the healthcare system to work towards reducing inequalities in care and eliminating discrimination. The act sets out that every patient has the right to be treated as an individual, and with fairness, respect and dignity. The act confers protection to 9 characteristics: age, race, sex, gender reassignment status, disability, religion/belief, sexual orientation, marriage/civil partnership status and pregnancy/maternity. In principle, patients should have equal access to care regardless of their status under these 9 characteristics. A common example is ensuring that clinical areas are able to be accessed by those with mobility difficulties.

Duty of Candour

Doctors have for many years had a professional duty of candour, which means that they have the responsibility to be open and honest with patients when something goes wrong with their care or treatment that causes, or has the potential to cause, harm or distress. This is outlined in the General Medical Council's *Good Medical Practice* guidance for doctors. The professional duty of candour gives you as a clinician the responsibility to tell the patient (or if appropriate the patient's advocate, carer or family) when something has gone wrong, to apologize for what has happened and to explain as well as possible the short and long term sequelae of what has happened. Clinicians are also required to be open and honest with their colleagues, employers and regulators, including taking part in incident reviews and investigations where necessary.

On the 27th November 2014 a new statutory duty of candour was introduced for all NHS bodies in England. This was widened to include any care provider registered with the Care Quality Commission (CQC) from the 1st April 2015. The statutory duty of candour gives care organizations a legal obligation to be honest and open with patients when something goes wrong with their care. A brief summary of the obligations of the statutory duty of candour is given:

- Care organizations have a general duty to act in an open and transparent way
- The statutory duty applies to organizations (but individuals should remember that they have a professional duty of candour to patients)
- As soon as is reasonably practical after a notifiable patient safety incident occurs, the organization must tell the patient (or their representative) about it in person

- A full explanation of what is known at the time (including what further investigations will be carried out) should be given to the patient, including an apology- a written record must be kept of the notification to the patient.
- An apology does not imply an admission of legal liability
- Reasonable support must be given to the patient, e.g. providing an interpreter
- Once the patient has been told in person about the incident, the organization should provide the patient with a written summary of the discussion

Under the statutory duty of candour, a notifiable patient safety incident has a specific meaning. It applies to incidents where a patient suffered (or could suffer) unintended harm that results in death, severe harm, moderate harm or prolonged psychological harm (for more than 28 days continuously). Moderate harm refers to 'any patient safety incident that resulted in a moderate increase in treatment and which caused significant but not permanent harm to one or more persons'.

The threshold for notification under the statutory duty can sometimes be an area of debate, but a doctor's professional duty to be candid with patients is an easier obligation to understand as this applies to any harm or distress caused to a patient.

In the Part 3 examination, the duty of candour is most likely to come up in the context of a communication skills clinical assessment task. Scenarios during which knowledge of the duty of candour may be tested may include discussing a post-operative complication with a patient, or breaking the news of an intra-uterine death in the context of concerns regarding poor care. It is important to remember the principles of good communication when tackling a clinical assessment task relating to duty of candour, as this plays a pivotal role in how you will come across to a patient in this type of difficult conversation. A sensitive and empathetic approach will go a long way towards helping the patient feel supported during what is effectively a breaking bad news situation. In reality, the team member who will provide the explanation and apology for a moderate or severe harm under the statutory duty of candour is likely to be the consultant, however the ethical principles of the professional duty of candour are the same for all harms, regardless of severity, and you may be given a scenario involving a lesser degree of harm. It is important to be aware of the threshold for and obligations of the statutory duty, as this is an issue that could be asked about.

Some tips for approaching a duty of candour scenario are given:

- The role player may be given instructions to behave in an emotionally charged manner. Remain calm, keep your posture open and not defensive, speak slowly and clearly, maintain good eye contact, and listen to what the role player says to you
- Ask the role player if they would like someone with them to support them. Clearly in a clinical assessment task there will just be the patient alone- but it looks more professional if you offer this
- Begin by giving a clear and accurate account of what has happened to the patient. Avoid medical jargon. Explain (if applicable) what the consequences are likely to be
- Respond honestly to any questions; if you do not have the answers, say so.
- An apology for the harm is crucial- this does not mean that you are taking personal responsibility for what has gone wrong
- Empathize and acknowledge any anger/emotional upset that the patient displays
- Explain that the safety incident will be investigated and that the patient will be contacted once this investigation is complete

Further reading

General Medical Council: Good Medical Practice. http://www.gmc-uk.org/guidance/

When things go wrong—The professional duty of candour, General Medical Council, UK. http://www.gmc-uk.org/guidance/ethical_guidance/27233.asp

Index

Notes: Tables, figures, and boxes are indicated by an italic *t*, *f*, and *b* following the page number.

D

H

I

R

S

T

U

V

W

Z